CDT 2024

Current Dental Terminology

ADA® *ADA is the official and definitive source for CDT.*

Book ISBN: 978-1-68447-201-7

E-book ISBN: 978-1-68447-202-4

ADA Product No.: J024

Acknowledgments

The American Dental Association's Council on Dental Benefit Programs, Practice Institute Center for Dental Benefits Coding and Quality, and Product Development are responsible for the technical content and format of this publication.

Principal staff contributions to *CDT 2024: Current Dental Terminology* were made by:

Dr. Krishna Aravamudhan, Vice President, Practice Institute

Afton Dunsmoor, Manager, Dental Codes Maintenance and Development, CDBCQ

Rebekah Fiehn, Director, Dental Codes Maintenance and Development, CDBCQ

Frank Pokorny, MBA, FACD (hon.), Senior Manager, Dental Codes Maintenance and Development, CDBCQ

Stacy Starnes, Coordinator, CDBCQ

Caitlin Wilson, Manager, Product Development

Pamela Woolf, Director, Product Development

CDT 2024
Current Dental Terminology

Table of Contents

Preface

Introduction

This reference manual, published by the ADA, contains the *Code on Dental Procedures and Nomenclature* (CDT Code) version that is effective for services provided on or after January 1, 2024 through December 31, 2024.

In August 2000, the CDT Code was designated by the federal government as the national terminology for reporting dental services on claims submitted to third-party payers, in accordance with authority granted by the Health Insurance Portability and Accountability Act of 1996 (HIPAA).

The ADA's Council on Dental Benefit Programs is responsible for maintaining the CDT Code in accordance with ADA Bylaws and policy and applicable federal regulations. *Current Dental Terminology* (CDT) technical content is developed by staff in the ADA Practice Institute's Center for Dental Benefits Coding and Quality, while responsibility for this manual's printing, pricing, and distribution falls to the ADA's Department of Product Development and Sales.

Should you have any recommendations for CDT Code additions, revisions, or deletions, information concerning the code set's maintenance process is available online at *ADA.org/cdt*.

For questions about dental procedure coding or claim submission the ADA provides the following support options:

1. Email *msc@ADA.org* or call the member service center at 800.947.4746. Support is available from 8:30 a.m. to 6:00 p.m. Central Time, Monday through Friday.

2. Email *dentalcode@ADA.org*; written inquiries will be responded to within two business days.

3. Online coding education guides, by topic and by CDT code, available for download at *ADA.org/cdt* and *ADA.org/publications/cdt/coding-education*

4. The *CDT Coding Companion;* visit *ADAStore.org* or call 800.947.4746.

For general information about, or to pursue CDT Code licensing, visit *ADA.org/CDTlicensing.* In addition to information about licensing, this site contains the questionnaire that must be completed as the first step of the licensing process.

For any questions regarding pricing or purchasing additional copies of CDT, visit ADAStore.org or call 800.947.4746. If you are ordering 25 or more copies or if you are ordering for an educational institution, please email *SpecialOrdersPDS@ADA.org* to request a quote.

Components of a Dental Procedure Code Entry

Every procedure in the CDT Code must have the first two of the following three components:

1. Procedure Code

A five-character alphanumeric code beginning with the letter "D" that identifies a specific dental procedure. A Procedure Code cannot be changed or abbreviated.

2. Nomenclature

The written title of a Procedure Code. Nomenclature may be abbreviated when printed on claim forms or other documents that are subject to space limitation. Any such abbreviation does not constitute a change to the Nomenclature.

3. Descriptor

A written narrative that further defines the nature and intended use of a single Procedure Code, or group of such codes. A Descriptor, when present, follows the applicable Procedure Code and its Nomenclature. Descriptors that apply to a series of Procedure Codes precede that series of codes.

Preface

Categories of Service (Also Known as Procedure Code Groups)

In this manual, the CDT Code is presented in several groupings identified as categories of service and, within each, one or more subcategories (etc.) to organize the content. Several of these named divisions are followed by narrative information that is applicable to all procedure codes within that division.

The following table illustrates the highest-level groupings, known as Categories of Service:

Category of Service
I. Diagnostic
II. Preventive
III. Restorative
IV. Endodontics
V. Periodontics
VI. Prosthodontics, removable
VII. Maxillofacial Prosthetics
VIII. Implant Services
IX. Prosthodontics, fixed
X. Oral & Maxillofacial Surgery
XI. Orthodontics
XII. Adjunctive General Services
XIII. Sleep Apnea Services

These categories, and subcategories (et al.) within, organize the CDT Code.
This structure, and the manual's alphabetic and numeric indices, are aids to finding the applicable code to document and report a procedure delivered to a patient.

> **Note:** Dental procedure codes are not always listed in numeric order. The reason is that existing numeric sequences within a named division often do not have unassigned codes available within the sequence when a CDT code is added.

Using the CDT Code

The following points should prove helpful when using the CDT Code for recording services provided on the patient record and when reporting procedures on a paper or electronic claim submission.

1. The presence of a CDT code **does not mean** that the procedure is:
   a. endorsed by any entity or is considered a standard of care
   b. covered or reimbursed by a dental benefits plan

2. General practitioners, specialists, and other individuals **may report any of the listed CDT codes** as long as they are delivering procedures and services within the scope of their state law.

3. CDT codes that require inclusion of a narrative description on the claim have the words "by report" in their nomenclature.

4. "Unspecified... procedure, by report" codes are used when, in the opinion of the dentist, there is no other CDT Code entry that accurately describes the services provided to the patient.

5. Documentation of services provided may necessitate selection of CDT codes from different categories of service. Two illustrative scenarios follow. Section 4 "Alphabetic Index to the CDT Code" (starting on page 143) will also help you locate the page number for an applicable procedure code.

Preface

Scenario Description	Procedure Delivered	Category of Service
	Radiographs	Diagnostic
1. Implant Case – Four-unit Fixed Partial Denture	Implant body placement	Implant Services
	Implant supported retainers	
	Pontics	Prosthodontics, fixed
2. Orthodontic Case – Treatment Planning	Pre-treatment examination	Orthodontics
	Radiographs	Diagnostic
	Diagnostic casts	
	Case presentation	Adjunctive General Services

Required Statement

If there is more than one code in this edition that consists of a procedure and a dentist submits a claim under one of these codes, the payor may process the claim under any of these codes that is consistent with the payor's reimbursement policy.

Section 1

Code on Dental Procedures and Nomenclature (CDT Code)

The current version of the *Code on Dental Procedures and Nomenclature* (CDT Code) that follows is effective for the calendar year 2024. There are a number of changes from the prior version that, where applicable, are identified by the following symbols:

- ● New procedure code
- ▲ Substantive revision to a nomenclature or descriptor
- \# Editorial

Dental procedure codes that are no longer valid are not present. Section 2 contains the summary of all additions, revisions, and deletions effective January 1, 2024.

Please note that when a code's nomenclature includes a "by report" notation, a narrative explaining the treatment provided must be included with the claim submission.

Classification of Materials

Names of dental materials are included in numerous procedure nomenclatures within several Categories of Service (e.g., Restorative; Prosthodontics, fixed; etc.). The following list of dental materials is included in the CDT Code **solely to aid selection** of a procedure code applicable to the service provided.

- **Classification of Metals (Source: ADA Council on Scientific Affairs, 2003)**
  The noble metal classification system supports reporting various alloys used in dentistry. The alloys are defined on the basis of the percentage of metal content.

Classification	Requirement
High Noble Alloys	Noble Metal Content ≥ 60% (gold+ platinum group*) and gold ≥ 40%
Titanium and Titanium Alloys	Titanium ≥ 85%
Noble Alloys	Noble Metal Content ≥ 25% (gold + platinum group*)
Predominantly Base Alloys	Noble Metal Content < 25% (gold + platinum group*)

* metals of the platinum group are platinum, palladium, rhodium, iridium, osmium, and ruthenium

- **Porcelain/ceramic**
  Refers to materials containing predominantly inorganic refractory compounds including porcelains, glasses, ceramics, and glass-ceramics.

- **Resin**
  Refers to any resin-based composite, including fiber or ceramic reinforced polymer compounds, and glass ionomers.

I. Diagnostic

Clinical Oral Evaluations

The codes in this section recognize the cognitive skills necessary for patient evaluation. The collection and recording of some data and components of the dental examination may be delegated; however, the evaluation, which includes diagnosis and treatment planning, is the responsibility of the dentist. As with all ADA procedure codes, there is no distinction made between the evaluations provided by general practitioners and specialists. Report additional diagnostic or definitive procedures separately.

D0120 **periodic oral evaluation – established patient**
An evaluation performed on a patient of record to determine any changes in the patient's dental and medical health status since a previous comprehensive or periodic evaluation. This includes an oral cancer evaluation, periodontal screening where indicated, and may require interpretation of information acquired through additional diagnostic procedures. The findings are discussed with the patient. Report additional diagnostic procedures separately.

D0140 **limited oral evaluation – problem focused**
An evaluation limited to a specific oral health problem or complaint. This may require interpretation of information acquired through additional diagnostic procedures. Report additional diagnostic procedures separately. Definitive procedures may be required on the same date as the evaluation.

Typically, patients receiving this type of evaluation present with a specific problem and/or dental emergencies, trauma, acute infections, etc.

D0145 **oral evaluation for a patient under three years of age and counseling with primary caregiver**
Diagnostic services performed for a child under the age of three, preferably within the first six months of the eruption of the first primary tooth, including recording the oral and physical health history, evaluation of caries susceptibility, development of an appropriate preventive oral health regimen and communication with and counseling of the child's parent, legal guardian and/or primary caregiver.

D0150 **comprehensive oral evaluation – new or established patient**

Used by a general dentist and/or a specialist when evaluating a patient comprehensively. This applies to new patients; established patients who have had a significant change in health conditions or other unusual circumstances, by report, or established patients who have been absent from active treatment for three or more years. It is a thorough evaluation and recording of the extraoral and intraoral hard and soft tissues.

It may require interpretation of information acquired through additional diagnostic procedures. Additional diagnostic procedures should be reported separately.

This includes an evaluation for oral cancer, the evaluation and recording of the patient's dental and medical history and a general health assessment. It may include the evaluation and recording of dental caries, missing or unerupted teeth, restorations, existing prostheses, occlusal relationships, periodontal conditions (including periodontal screening and/or charting), hard and soft tissue anomalies, etc.

D0160 **detailed and extensive oral evaluation – problem focused, by report**

A detailed and extensive problem focused evaluation entails extensive diagnostic and cognitive modalities based on the findings of a comprehensive oral evaluation. Integration of more extensive diagnostic modalities to develop a treatment plan for a specific problem is required. The condition requiring this type of evaluation should be described and documented.

Examples of conditions requiring this type of evaluation may include dentofacial anomalies, complicated perio-prosthetic conditions, complex temporomandibular dysfunction, facial pain of unknown origin, conditions requiring multi-disciplinary consultation, etc.

D0170 **re-evaluation – limited, problem focused (established patient; not post-operative visit)**

Assessing the status of a previously existing condition. For example:
- a traumatic injury where no treatment was rendered but patient needs follow-up monitoring;
- evaluation for undiagnosed continuing pain;
- soft tissue lesion requiring follow-up evaluation.

D0171 **re-evaluation – post-operative office visit**

D0180   comprehensive periodontal evaluation – new or established patient
This procedure is indicated for patients showing signs or symptoms of periodontal disease and for patients with risk factors such as smoking or diabetes. It includes evaluation of periodontal conditions, probing and charting, an evaluation for oral cancer, the evaluation and recording of the patient's dental and medical history and general health assessment. It may include the evaluation and recording of dental caries, missing or unerupted teeth, restorations, and occlusal relationships.

Pre-diagnostic Services

D0190   screening of a patient
A screening, including state or federally mandated screenings, to determine an individual's need to be seen by a dentist for diagnosis.

D0191   assessment of a patient
A limited clinical inspection that is performed to identify possible signs of oral or systemic disease, malformation, or injury, and the potential need for referral for diagnosis and treatment.

Diagnostic Imaging

Should be taken only for clinical reasons as determined by the patient's dentist. Should be of diagnostic quality and properly identified and dated. Is a part of the patient's clinical record and the original images should be retained by the dentist. Originals should not be used to fulfill requests made by patients or third-parties for copies of records.

Image Capture with Interpretation

D0210   intraoral – comprehensive series of radiographic images
A radiographic survey of the whole mouth intended to display the crowns and roots of all teeth, periapical areas, interproximal areas and alveolar bone including edentulous areas.

D0220   intraoral – periapical first radiographic image

D0230   intraoral – periapical each additional radiographic image

D0240   intraoral – occlusal radiographic image

D0250   extra-oral – 2D projection radiographic image created using a stationary radiation source, and detector
These images include, but are not limited to: Lateral Skull; Posterior-Anterior Skull; Submentovertex; Waters; Reverse Tomes; Oblique Mandibular Body; Lateral Ramus.

D0251 **extra-oral posterior dental radiographic image**
Image limited to exposure of complete posterior teeth in both dental arches. This is a unique image that is not derived from another image.

D0270 **bitewing – single radiographic image**

D0272 **bitewings – two radiographic images**

D0273 **bitewings – three radiographic images**

D0274 **bitewings – four radiographic images**

D0277 **vertical bitewings – 7 to 8 radiographic images**
This does not constitute a full mouth intraoral radiographic series.

D0310 **sialography**

D0320 **temporomandibular joint arthrogram, including injection**

D0321 **other temporomandibular joint radiographic images, by report**

D0322 **tomographic survey**

D0330 **panoramic radiographic image**

D0340 **2D cephalometric radiographic image – acquisition, measurement and analysis**
Image of the head made using a cephalostat to standardize anatomic positioning, and with reproducible x-ray beam geometry.

D0350 **2D oral/facial photographic image obtained intra-orally or extra-orally**

D0364 **cone beam CT capture and interpretation with limited field of view – less than one whole jaw**

D0365 **cone beam CT capture and interpretation with field of view of one full dental arch – mandible**

D0366 **cone beam CT capture and interpretation with field of view of one full dental arch – maxilla, with or without cranium**

D0367 **cone beam CT capture and interpretation with field of view of both jaws; with or without cranium**

D0368 **cone beam CT capture and interpretation for TMJ series including two or more exposures**

D0369 **maxillofacial MRI capture and interpretation**

  ● new procedure code ▲ revision to a nomenclature or descriptor # editorial

D0370   **maxillofacial ultrasound capture and interpretation**

D0371   **sialoendoscopy capture and interpretation**

D0372   **intraoral tomosynthesis – comprehensive series of radiographic images**
A radiographic survey of the whole mouth intended to display the crowns and roots of all teeth, periapical areas, interproximal areas and alveolar bone including edentulous areas.

D0373   **intraoral tomosynthesis – bitewing radiographic image**

D0374   **intraoral tomosynthesis – periapical radiographic image**

D0801   **3D dental surface scan – direct**

D0802   **3D dental surface scan – indirect**
A surface scan of a diagnostic cast.

D0803   **3D facial surface scan – direct**

D0804   **3D facial surface scan – indirect**
A surface scan of constructed facial features.

Image Capture Only

Capture by a Practitioner not associated with Interpretation and Report

D0380   **cone beam CT image capture with limited field of view – less than one whole jaw**

D0381   **cone beam CT image capture with field of view of one full dental arch – mandible**

D0382   **cone beam CT image capture with field of view of one full dental arch – maxilla, with or without cranium**

D0383   **cone beam CT image capture with field of view of both jaws, with or without cranium**

D0384   **cone beam CT image capture for TMJ series including two or more exposures**

D0385   **maxillofacial MRI image capture**

D0386   **maxillofacial ultrasound image capture**

Section 1: Code on Dental Procedures and Nomenclature

D0387   **intraoral tomosynthesis – comprehensive series of radiographic images – image capture only**
A radiographic survey of the whole mouth intended to display the crowns and roots of all teeth, periapical areas, interproximal areas and alveolar bone including edentulous areas.

D0388   **intraoral tomosynthesis – bitewing radiographic image – image capture only**

D0389   **intraoral tomosynthesis – periapical radiographic image – image capture only**

D0701   **panoramic radiographic image – image capture only**

D0702   **2-D cephalometric radiographic image – image capture only**

D0703   **2-D oral/facial photographic image obtained intra-orally or extra-orally – image capture only**

D0705   **extra-oral posterior dental radiographic image – image capture only**
Image limited to exposure of complete posterior teeth in both dental arches. This is a unique image that is not derived from another image.

D0706   **intraoral – occlusal radiographic image – image capture only**

D0707   **intraoral – periapical radiographic image – image capture only**

D0708   **intraoral – bitewing radiographic image – image capture only**
Image axis may be horizontal or vertical.

D0709   **intraoral – comprehensive series of radiographic images – image capture only**
A radiographic survey of the whole mouth intended to display the crowns and roots of all teeth, periapical areas, interproximal areas and alveolar bone including edentulous areas.

Interpretation and Report Only

Interpretation and report by a practitioner not associated with image capture.

D0391   **interpretation of diagnostic image by a practitioner not associated with capture of the image, including report**

● new procedure code   ▲ revision to a nomenclature or descriptor   # editorial

Post Processing of Image or Image Sets

D0393 **virtual treatment simulation using 3D image volume or surface scan**
Virtual simulation of treatment including, but not limited to, dental implant placement, prosthetic reconstruction, orthognathic surgery and orthodontic tooth movement.

D0394 **digital subtraction of two or more images or image volumes of the same modality**
To demonstrate changes that have occurred over time.

D0395 **fusion of two or more 3D image volumes of one or more modalities**

• **D0396** **3D printing of a 3D dental surface scan**
3D printing of a 3D dental surface scan to obtain a physical model.

Tests and Examinations

D0411 **HbA1c in-office point of service testing**

D0412 **blood glucose level test – in-office using a glucose meter**
This procedure provides an immediate finding of a patient's blood glucose level at the time of sample collection for the point-of-service analysis.

D0414 **laboratory processing of microbial specimen to include culture and sensitivity studies, preparation and transmission of written report**

D0415 **collection of microorganisms for culture and sensitivity**

D0416 **viral culture**
A diagnostic test to identify viral organisms, most often herpes virus.

D0417 **collection and preparation of saliva sample for laboratory diagnostic testing**

D0418 **analysis of saliva sample**
Chemical or biological analysis of saliva sample for diagnostic purposes.

D0419 **assessment of salivary flow by measurement**
This procedure is for identification of low salivary flow in patients at risk for hyposalivation and xerostomia, as well as effectiveness of pharmacological agents used to stimulate saliva production.

D0422 **collection and preparation of genetic sample material for laboratory analysis and report**

D0423 **genetic test for susceptibility to diseases – specimen analysis**
Certified laboratory analysis to detect specific genetic variations associated with increased susceptibility for diseases.

D0425 **caries susceptibility tests**
Not to be used for carious dentin staining.

D0431 **adjunctive pre-diagnostic test that aids in detection of mucosal abnormalities including premalignant and malignant lesions, not to include cytology or biopsy procedures**

D0460 **pulp vitality tests**
Includes multiple teeth and contra lateral comparison(s), as indicated.

D0470 **diagnostic casts**
Also known as diagnostic models or study models.

D0600 **non-ionizing diagnostic procedure capable of quantifying, monitoring, and recording changes in structure of enamel, dentin, and cementum**

D0601 **caries risk assessment and documentation, with a finding of low risk**
Using recognized assessment tools.

D0602 **caries risk assessment and documentation, with a finding of moderate risk**
Using recognized assessment tools.

D0603 **caries risk assessment and documentation, with a finding of high risk**
Using recognized assessment tools.

D0604 **antigen testing for a public health related pathogen, including coronavirus**

D0605 **antibody testing for a public health related pathogen, including coronavirus**

D0606 **molecular testing for a public health related pathogen, including coronavirus**

Oral Pathology Laboratory

These procedures do not include collection of the tissue sample, which is documented separately.

D0472 **accession of tissue, gross examination, preparation and transmission of written report**
To be used in reporting architecturally intact tissue obtained by invasive means.

D0473 **accession of tissue, gross and microscopic examination, preparation and transmission of written report**
To be used in reporting architecturally intact tissue obtained by invasive means.

D0474 **accession of tissue, gross and microscopic examination, including assessment of surgical margins for presence of disease, preparation and transmission of written report**
To be used in reporting architecturally intact tissue obtained by invasive means.

D0480 **accession of exfoliative cytologic smears, microscopic examination, preparation and transmission of written report**
To be used in reporting disaggregated, non-transepithelial cell cytology sample via mild scraping of the oral mucosa.

D0486 **laboratory accession of transepithelial cytologic sample, microscopic examination, preparation and transmission of written report**
Analysis, and written report of findings, of cytological sample of disaggregated transepithelial cells.

D0475 **decalcification procedure**
Procedure in which hard tissue is processed in order to allow sectioning and subsequent microscopic examination.

D0476 **special stains for microorganisms**
Procedure in which additional stains are applied to biopsy or surgical specimen in order to identify microorganisms.

D0477 **special stains, not for microorganisms**
Procedure in which additional stains are applied to a biopsy or surgical specimen in order to identify such things as melanin, mucin, iron, glycogen, etc.

D0478 **immunohistochemical stains**
A procedure in which specific antibody based reagents are applied to tissue samples in order to facilitate diagnosis.

D0479 **tissue in–situ hybridization, including interpretation**
A procedure which allows for the identification of nucleic acids, DNA and RNA, in the tissue sample in order to aid in the diagnosis of microorganisms and tumors.

D0481 **electron microscopy**

D0482 **direct immunofluorescence**
A technique used to identify immunoreactants which are localized to the patient's skin or mucous membranes.

D0483 **indirect immunofluorescence**
A technique used to identify circulating immunoreactants.

D0484 **consultation on slides prepared elsewhere**
A service provided in which microscopic slides of a biopsy specimen prepared at another laboratory are evaluated to aid in the diagnosis of a difficult case or to offer a consultative opinion at the patient's request. The findings are delivered by written report.

D0485 **consultation, including preparation of slides from biopsy material supplied by referring source**
A service that requires the consulting pathologist to prepare the slides as well as render a written report. The slides are evaluated to aid in the diagnosis of a difficult case or to offer a consultative opinion at the patient's request.

D0502 **other oral pathology procedures, by report**

D0999 **unspecified diagnostic procedure, by report**
Used for a procedure that is not adequately described by a code. Describe the procedure.

II. Preventive

Dental Prophylaxis

D1110 **prophylaxis – adult**
Removal of plaque, calculus and stains from the tooth structures and implants in the permanent and transitional dentition. It is intended to control local irritational factors.

D1120 **prophylaxis – child**
Removal of plaque, calculus and stains from the tooth structures and implants in the primary and transitional dentition. It is intended to control local irritational factors.

Topical Fluoride Treatment (Office Procedure)

Prescription strength fluoride product designed solely for use in the dental office, delivered to the dentition under the direct supervision of a dental professional. Fluoride must be applied separately from prophylaxis paste.

D1206 **topical application of fluoride varnish**

D1208 **topical application of fluoride – excluding varnish**

Other Preventive Services

● **D1301** **immunization counseling**
A review of a patient's vaccine and medical history, discussion of the vaccine benefits, risks, and consequences of not obtaining the vaccine. Counseling also includes a discussion of questions and concerns the patient, family, or caregiver may have and suggestions on where the patient can obtain the vaccine.

D1310 **nutritional counseling for control of dental disease**
Counseling on food selection and dietary habits as a part of treatment and control of periodontal disease and caries.

D1320 **tobacco counseling for the control and prevention of oral disease**
Tobacco prevention and cessation services reduce patient risks of developing tobacco-related oral diseases and conditions and improves prognosis for certain dental therapies.

Section 1: Code on Dental Procedures and Nomenclature

D1321 **counseling for the control and prevention of adverse oral, behavioral, and systemic health effects associated with high-risk substance use**
Counseling services may include patient education about adverse oral, behavioral, and systemic effects associated with high-risk substance use and administration routes. This includes ingesting, injecting, inhaling and vaping. Substances used in a high-risk manner may include but are not limited to alcohol, opioids, nicotine, cannabis, methamphetamine and other pharmaceuticals or chemicals.

D1330 **oral hygiene instructions**
This may include instructions for home care. Examples include tooth brushing technique, flossing, and use of special oral hygiene aids.

D1351 **sealant – per tooth**
Mechanically and/or chemically prepared enamel surface sealed to prevent decay.

D1353 **sealant repair – per tooth**

D1352 **preventive resin restoration in a moderate to high caries risk patient – permanent tooth**
Conservative restoration of an active cavitated lesion in a pit or fissure that does not extend into dentin; includes placement of a sealant in any radiating non-carious fissures or pits.

D1354 **application of caries arresting medicament – per tooth**
Conservative treatment of an active, non-symptomatic carious lesion by topical application of a caries arresting or inhibiting medicament and without mechanical removal of sound tooth structure.

D1355 **caries preventive medicament application – per tooth**
For primary prevention or remineralization. Medicaments applied do not include topical fluorides.

Space Maintenance (Passive Appliances)

Passive appliances are designed to prevent tooth movement.

D1510 **space maintainer – fixed, unilateral – per quadrant**
Excludes a distal shoe space maintainer.

D1516 **space maintainer – fixed – bilateral, maxillary**

D1517 **space maintainer – fixed – bilateral, mandibular**

D1520   **space maintainer – removable, unilateral – per quadrant**

D1526   **space maintainer – removable – bilateral, maxillary**

D1527   **space maintainer – removable – bilateral, mandibular**

D1551   **re-cement or re-bond bilateral space maintainer – maxillary**

D1552   **re-cement or re-bond bilateral space maintainer – mandibular**

D1553   **re-cement or re-bond unilateral space maintainer – per quadrant**

D1556   **removal of fixed unilateral space maintainer – per quadrant**

D1557   **removal of fixed bilateral space maintainer – maxillary**

D1558   **removal of fixed bilateral space maintainer – mandibular**

Space Maintainers

D1575   **distal shoe space maintainer – fixed, unilateral – per quadrant**
Fabrication and delivery of fixed appliance extending subgingivally and distally to guide the eruption of the first permanent molar. Does not include ongoing follow-up or adjustments, or replacement appliances, once the tooth has erupted.

Vaccinations

D1701   **Pfizer-BioNTech Covid-19 vaccine administration – first dose**
SARSCOV2 COVID-19 VAC mRNA 30mcg/0.3mL IM DOSE 1

D1702   **Pfizer-BioNTech Covid-19 vaccine administration – second dose**
SARSCOV2 COVID-19 VAC mRNA 30mcg/0.3mL IM DOSE 2

D1703   **Moderna Covid-19 vaccine administration – first dose**
SARSCOV2 COVID-19 VAC mRNA 100mcg/0.5mL IM DOSE 1

D1704   **Moderna Covid-19 vaccine administration – second dose**
SARSCOV2 COVID-19 VAC mRNA 100mcg/0.5mL IM DOSE 2

D1705   **AstraZeneca Covid-19 vaccine administration – first dose**
SARSCOV2 COVID-19 VAC rS-ChAdOx1 5x1010 VP/.5mL IM DOSE 1

D1706   **AstraZeneca Covid-19 vaccine administration – second dose**
SARSCOV2 COVID-19 VAC rS-ChAdOx1 5x1010 VP/.5mL IM DOSE 2

D1707   **Janssen Covid-19 vaccine administration**
SARSCOV2 COVID-19 VAC Ad26 5x1010 VP/.5mL IM SINGLE DOSE

D1708 **Pfizer-BioNTech Covid-19 vaccine administration – third dose**
SARSCOV2 COVID-19 VAC mRNA 30mcg/0.3mL IM DOSE 3

D1709 **Pfizer-BioNTech Covid-19 vaccine administration – booster dose**
SARSCOV2 COVID-19 VAC mRNA 30mcg/0.3mL IM DOSE BOOSTER

D1710 **Moderna Covid-19 vaccine administration – third dose**
SARSCOV2 COVID-19 VAC mRNA 100mcg/0.5mL IM DOSE 3

D1711 **Moderna Covid-19 vaccine administration – booster dose**
SARSCOV2 COVID-19 VAC mRNA 50mcg/0.25mL IM DOSE BOOSTER

D1712 **Janssen Covid-19 vaccine administration – booster dose**
SARSCOV2 COVID-19 VAC Ad26 5x1010 VP/.5mL IM DOSE BOOSTER

D1713 **Pfizer-BioNTech Covid-19 vaccine administration tris-sucrose pediatric – first dose**
SARSCOV2 COVID-19 VAC mRNA 10mcg/0.2mL tris-sucrose IM DOSE 1

D1714 **Pfizer-BioNTech Covid-19 vaccine administration tris-sucrose pediatric – second dose**
SARSCOV2 COVID-19 VAC mRNA 10mcg/0.2mL tris-sucrose IM DOSE 2

D1781 **vaccine administration – human papillomavirus – Dose 1**
Gardasil 9 0.5mL intramuscular vaccine injection.

D1782 **vaccine administration – human papillomavirus – Dose 2**
Gardasil 9 0.5mL intramuscular vaccine injection.

D1783 **vaccine administration – human papillomavirus – Dose 3**
Gardasil 9 0.5mL intramuscular vaccine injection.

D1999 **unspecified preventive procedure, by report**
Used for a procedure that is not adequately described by a code.
Describe the procedure.

III. Restorative

Local anesthesia is usually considered to be part of Restorative procedures.

Explanation of Restorations

Location	Number of Surfaces	Characteristics
Anterior	1	Placed on one of the following five surface classifications – Mesial, Distal, Incisal, Lingual, or Facial (or Labial).
	2	Placed, without interruption, on two of the five surface classifications – e.g., Mesial-Lingual.
	3	Placed, without interruption, on three of the five surface classifications – e.g., Lingual-Mesial-Facial (or Labial).
	4 or more	Placed, without interruption, on four or more of the five surface classifications – e.g., Mesial-Incisal-Lingual-Facial (or Labial).
Posterior	1	Placed on one of the following five surface classifications – Mesial, Distal, Occlusal, Lingual, or Buccal.
	2	Placed, without interruption, on two of the five surface classifications – e.g., Mesial-Occlusal.
	3	Placed, without interruption, on three of the five surface classifications – e.g., Lingual-Occlusal-Distal.
	4 or more	Placed, without interruption, on four or more of the five surface classifications – e.g., Mesial-Occlusal-Lingual-Distal.

Note: Tooth surfaces are reported on the HIPAA standard electronic dental transaction and the ADA Dental Claim Form using the letters in the following table.

Surface	Code
Buccal	B
Distal	D
Facial (or Labial)	F
Incisal	I
Lingual	L
Mesial	M
Occlusal	O

Section 1: Code on Dental Procedures and Nomenclature

Amalgam Restorations (Including Polishing)

Tooth preparation, all adhesives (including amalgam bonding agents), liners and bases are included as part of the restoration. If pins are used, they should be reported separately (see D2951).

D2140 **amalgam – one surface, primary or permanent**

D2150 **amalgam – two surfaces, primary or permanent**

D2160 **amalgam – three surfaces, primary or permanent**

D2161 **amalgam – four or more surfaces, primary or permanent**

Resin-Based Composite Restorations – Direct

Resin-based composite refers to a broad category of materials including but not limited to composites. May include bonded composite, light-cured composite, etc. Tooth preparation, acid etching, adhesives (including resin bonding agents), liners and bases, and curing are included as part of the restoration. Glass ionomers, when used as restorations, should be reported with these codes. If pins are used, they should be reported separately (see D2951).

D2330 **resin-based composite – one surface, anterior**

D2331 **resin-based composite – two surfaces, anterior**

D2332 **resin-based composite – three surfaces, anterior**

▲ **D2335** **resin-based composite – four or more surfaces (anterior)**

D2390 **resin-based composite crown, anterior**
  Full resin-based composite coverage of tooth.

D2391 **resin-based composite – one surface, posterior**
  Used to restore a carious lesion into the dentin or a deeply eroded area into the dentin. Not a preventive procedure.

D2392 **resin-based composite – two surfaces, posterior**

D2393 **resin-based composite – three surfaces, posterior**

D2394 **resin-based composite – four or more surfaces, posterior**

Gold Foil Restorations

D2410 **gold foil – one surface**

D2420 **gold foil – two surfaces**

D2430 **gold foil – three surfaces**

Inlay/Onlay Restorations

Inlay: An intra-coronal dental restoration, made outside the oral cavity to conform to the prepared cavity, which does not restore any cusp tips.

Onlay: A dental restoration made outside the oral cavity that covers one or more cusp tips and adjoining occlusal surfaces, but not the entire external surface.

D2510 inlay – metallic – one surface

D2520 inlay – metallic – two surfaces

D2530 inlay – metallic – three or more surfaces

D2542 onlay – metallic – two surfaces

D2543 onlay – metallic – three surfaces

D2544 onlay – metallic – four or more surfaces

Porcelain/ceramic inlays/onlays include all indirect ceramic and porcelain type inlays/onlays.

D2610 inlay – porcelain/ceramic – one surface

D2620 inlay – porcelain/ceramic – two surfaces

D2630 inlay – porcelain/ceramic – three or more surfaces

D2642 onlay – porcelain/ceramic – two surfaces

D2643 onlay – porcelain/ceramic – three surfaces

D2644 onlay – porcelain/ceramic – four or more surfaces

Resin-based composite inlays/onlays must utilize indirect technique.

D2650 inlay – resin-based composite – one surface

D2651 inlay – resin-based composite – two surfaces

D2652 inlay – resin-based composite – three or more surfaces

D2662 onlay – resin-based composite – two surfaces

D2663 onlay – resin-based composite – three surfaces

D2664 onlay – resin-based composite – four or more surfaces

Crowns – Single Restorations Only

D2710   **crown – resin-based composite (indirect)**

D2712   **crown – ¾ resin-based composite (indirect)**
This procedure does not include facial veneers.

D2720   **crown – resin with high noble metal**

D2721   **crown – resin with predominantly base metal**

D2722   **crown – resin with noble metal**

D2740   **crown – porcelain/ceramic**

D2750   **crown – porcelain fused to high noble metal**

D2751   **crown – porcelain fused to predominantly base metal**

D2752   **crown – porcelain fused to noble metal**

D2753   **crown – porcelain fused to titanium and titanium alloys**

D2780   **crown – ¾ cast high noble metal**

D2781   **crown – ¾ cast predominantly base metal**

D2782   **crown – ¾ cast noble metal**

D2783   **crown – ¾ porcelain/ceramic**
This procedure does not include facial veneers.

D2790   **crown – full cast high noble metal**

D2791   **crown – full cast predominantly base metal**

D2792   **crown – full cast noble metal**

D2794   **crown – titanium and titanium alloys**

D2799   **interim crown – further treatment or completion of diagnosis necessary prior to final impression**
Not to be used as a temporary crown for a routine prosthetic restoration.

Other Restorative Services

● **D2989**   **excavation of a tooth resulting in the determination of non-restorability**

D2990   **resin infiltration of incipient smooth surface lesions**
Placement of an infiltrating resin restoration for strengthening, stabilizing and/or limiting the progression of the lesion.

● **D2991** **application of hydroxyapatite regeneration medicament – per tooth**
Preparation of tooth surfaces and topical application of a scaffold to guide hydroxyapatite regeneration.

D2910 **re-cement or re-bond inlay, onlay, veneer or partial coverage restoration**

D2915 **re-cement or re-bond indirectly fabricated or prefabricated post and core**

D2920 **re-cement or re-bond crown**

D2921 **reattachment of tooth fragment, incisal edge or cusp**

D2929 **prefabricated porcelain/ceramic crown – primary tooth**

D2928 **prefabricated porcelain/ceramic crown – permanent tooth**

D2930 **prefabricated stainless steel crown – primary tooth**

D2931 **prefabricated stainless steel crown – permanent tooth**

D2932 **prefabricated resin crown**

D2933 **prefabricated stainless steel crown with resin window**
Open-face stainless steel crown with aesthetic resin facing or veneer.

D2934 **prefabricated esthetic coated stainless steel crown – primary tooth**
Stainless steel primary crown with exterior esthetic coating.

D2940 **protective restoration**
Direct placement of a restorative material to protect tooth and/or tissue form. This procedure may be used to relieve pain, promote healing, or prevent further deterioration. Not to be used for endodontic access closure, or as a base or liner under restoration.

D2941 **interim therapeutic restoration – primary dentition**
Placement of an adhesive restorative material following caries debridement by hand or other method for the management of early childhood caries. Not considered a definitive restoration.

D2949 **restorative foundation for an indirect restoration**
Placement of restorative material to yield a more ideal form, including elimination of undercuts.

D2950 **core buildup, including any pins when required**
Refers to building up of coronal structure when there is insufficient retention for a separate extracoronal restorative procedure. A core buildup is not a filler to eliminate any undercut, box form, or concave irregularity in a preparation.

D2951 **pin retention – per tooth, in addition to restoration**

D2952   **post and core in addition to crown, indirectly fabricated**
Post and core are custom fabricated as a single unit.

D2953   **each additional indirectly fabricated post – same tooth**
To be used with D2952.

D2954   **prefabricated post and core in addition to crown**
Core is built around a prefabricated post. This procedure includes the core material.

D2957   **each additional prefabricated post – same tooth**
To be used with D2954.

D2955   **post removal**

D2960   **labial veneer (resin laminate) – direct**
Refers to labial/facial direct resin bonded veneers.

D2961   **labial veneer (resin laminate) – indirect**
Refers to labial/facial indirect resin bonded veneers.

D2962   **labial veneer (porcelain laminate) – indirect**
Refers also to facial veneers that extend interproximally and/or cover the incisal edge. Porcelain/ceramic veneers presently include all ceramic and porcelain veneers.

D2971   **additional procedures to customize a crown to fit under an existing partial denture framework**
This procedure is in addition to the separate crown procedure documented with its own code.

D2975   **coping**
A thin covering of the coronal portion of a tooth, usually devoid of anatomic contour, that can be used as a definitive restoration.

● **D2976**   **band stabilization – per tooth**
A band, typically cemented around a molar tooth after a multi-surface restoration is placed, to add support and resistance to fracture until a patient is ready for the full cuspal coverage restoration.

D2980   **crown repair necessitated by restorative material failure**

D2981   **inlay repair necessitated by restorative material failure**

D2982   **onlay repair necessitated by restorative material failure**

D2983   **veneer repair necessitated by restorative material failure**

D2999   **unspecified restorative procedure, by report**
Use for a procedure that is not adequately described by a code. Describe the procedure.

IV. Endodontics

Local anesthesia is usually considered to be part of Endodontic procedures.

Pulp Capping

D3110 **pulp cap – direct (excluding final restoration)**
Procedure in which the exposed pulp is covered with a dressing or cement that protects the pulp and promotes healing and repair.

D3120 **pulp cap – indirect (excluding final restoration)**
Procedure in which the nearly exposed pulp is covered with a protective dressing to protect the pulp from additional injury and to promote healing and repair via formation of secondary dentin. This code is not to be used for bases and liners when all caries has been removed.

Pulpotomy

D3220 **therapeutic pulpotomy (excluding final restoration) – removal of pulp coronal to the dentinocemental junction and application of medicament**
Pulpotomy is the surgical removal of a portion of the pulp with the aim of maintaining the vitality of the remaining portion by means of an adequate dressing.
– To be performed on primary or permanent teeth.
– This is not to be construed as the first stage of root canal therapy.
– Not to be used for apexogenesis.

D3221 **pulpal debridement, primary and permanent teeth**
Pulpal debridement for the relief of acute pain prior to conventional root canal therapy. This procedure is not to be used when endodontic treatment is completed on the same day.

D3222 **partial pulpotomy for apexogenesis – permanent tooth with incomplete root development**
Removal of a portion of the pulp and application of a medicament with the aim of maintaining the vitality of the remaining portion to encourage continued physiological development and formation of the root. This procedure is not to be construed as the first stage of root canal therapy.

Endodontic Therapy on Primary Teeth

Endodontic therapy on primary teeth with succedaneous teeth and placement of resorbable filling. This includes pulpectomy, cleaning, and filling of canals with resorbable material.

D3230 **pulpal therapy (resorbable filling) – anterior, primary tooth (excluding final restoration)**
Primary incisors and cuspids.

D3240 **pulpal therapy (resorbable filling) – posterior, primary tooth (excluding final restoration)**
Primary first and second molars.

Endodontic Therapy (Including Treatment Plan, Clinical Procedures and Follow-Up Care)

Includes primary teeth without succedaneous teeth and permanent teeth. Complete root canal therapy; pulpectomy is part of root canal therapy.

Includes all appointments necessary to complete treatment; also includes intra-operative radiographs. Does not include diagnostic evaluation and necessary radiographs/diagnostic images.

D3310 **endodontic therapy, anterior tooth (excluding final restoration)**

D3320 **endodontic therapy, premolar tooth (excluding final restoration)**

D3330 **endodontic therapy, molar tooth (excluding final restoration)**

D3331 **treatment of root canal obstruction; non-surgical access**
In lieu of surgery, the formation of a pathway to achieve an apical seal without surgical intervention because of a non-negotiable root canal blocked by foreign bodies, including but not limited to separated instruments, broken posts or calcification of 50% or more of the length of the tooth root.

D3332 **incomplete endodontic therapy; inoperable, unrestorable or fractured tooth**
Considerable time is necessary to determine diagnosis and/or provide initial treatment before the fracture makes the tooth unretainable.

D3333 **internal root repair of perforation defects**
Non-surgical seal of perforation caused by resorption and/or decay but not iatrogenic by same provider.

Endodontic Retreatment

D3346   **retreatment of previous root canal therapy – anterior**

D3347   **retreatment of previous root canal therapy – premolar**

D3348   **retreatment of previous root canal therapy – molar**

Apexification/Recalcification

D3351   **apexification/recalcification – initial visit (apical closure/calcific repair of perforations, root resorption, etc.)**
Includes opening tooth, preparation of canal spaces, first placement of medication and necessary radiographs. (This procedure may include first phase of complete root canal therapy.)

D3352   **apexification/recalcification – interim medication replacement**
For visits in which the intra-canal medication is replaced with new medication. Includes any necessary radiographs.

D3353   **apexification/recalcification – final visit (includes completed root canal therapy – apical closure/calcific repair of perforations, root resorption, etc.)**
Includes removal of intra-canal medication and procedures necessary to place final root canal filling material including necessary radiographs. (This procedure includes last phase of complete root canal therapy.)

Pulpal Regeneration

D3355   **pulpal regeneration – initial visit**
Includes opening tooth, preparation of canal spaces, placement of medication.

D3356   **pulpal regeneration – interim medication replacement**

D3357   **pulpal regeneration – completion of treatment**
Does not include final restoration.

Section 1: Code on Dental Procedures and Nomenclature

Apicoectomy/Periradicular Services

Periradicular surgery is a term used to describe surgery to the root surface (e.g., apicoectomy), repair of a root perforation or resorptive defect, exploratory curettage to look for root fractures, removal of extruded filling materials or instruments, removal of broken root fragments, sealing of accessory canals, etc. This does not include retrograde filling material placement.

D3410   **apicoectomy – anterior**
For surgery on root of anterior tooth. Does not include placement of retrograde filling material.

D3421   **apicoectomy – premolar (first root)**
For surgery on one root of a premolar. Does not include placement of retrograde filling material. If more than one root is treated, see D3426.

D3425   **apicoectomy – molar (first root)**
For surgery on one root of a molar tooth. Does not include placement of retrograde filling material. If more than one root is treated, see D3426.

D3426   **apicoectomy (each additional root)**
Typically used for premolar and molar surgeries when more than one root is treated during the same procedure. This does not include retrograde filling material placement.

D3471   **surgical repair of root resorption – anterior**
For surgery on root of anterior tooth. Does not include placement of restoration.

D3472   **surgical repair of root resorption – premolar**
For surgery on root of premolar tooth. Does not include placement of restoration.

D3473   **surgical repair of root resorption – molar**
For surgery on root of molar tooth. Does not include placement of restoration.

D3501   **surgical exposure of root surface without apicoectomy or repair of root resorption – anterior**
Exposure of root surface followed by observation and surgical closure of the exposed area. Not to be used for or in conjunction with apicoectomy or repair of root resorption.

D3502 **surgical exposure of root surface without apicoectomy or repair of root resorption – premolar**
Exposure of root surface followed by observation and surgical closure of the exposed area. Not to be used for or in conjunction with apicoectomy or repair of root resorption.

D3503 **surgical exposure of root surface without apicoectomy or repair of root resorption – molar**
Exposure of root surface followed by observation and surgical closure of the exposed area. Not to be used for or in conjunction with apicoectomy or repair of root resorption.

D3428 **bone graft in conjunction with periradicular surgery – per tooth, single site**
Includes non-autogenous graft material.

D3429 **bone graft in conjunction with periradicular surgery – each additional contiguous tooth in the same surgical site**
Includes non-autogenous graft material.

D3430 **retrograde filling – per root**
For placement of retrograde filling material during periradicular surgery procedures. If more than one filling is placed in one root report as D3999 and describe.

D3431 **biologic materials to aid in soft and osseous tissue regeneration in conjunction with periradicular surgery**

D3432 **guided tissue regeneration, resorbable barrier, per site, in conjunction with periradicular surgery**

D3450 **root amputation – per root**
Root resection of a multi-rooted tooth while leaving the crown. If the crown is sectioned, see D3920.

D3460 **endodontic endosseous implant**
Placement of implant material, which extends from a pulpal space into the bone beyond the end of the root.

D3470 **intentional re-implantation (including necessary splinting)**
For the intentional removal, inspection and treatment of the root and replacement of a tooth into its own socket. This does not include necessary retrograde filling material placement.

Other Endodontic Procedures

D3910 **surgical procedure for isolation of tooth with rubber dam**

D3911 **intraorifice barrier**
Not to be used as a final restoration.

D3920 **hemisection (including any root removal), not including root canal therapy**
Includes separation of a multi-rooted tooth into separate sections containing the root and the overlying portion of the crown. It may also include the removal of one or more of those sections.

D3921 **decoronation or submergence of an erupted tooth**
Intentional removal of coronal tooth structure for preservation of root and surrounding bone.

D3950 **canal preparation and fitting of preformed dowel or post**
Should not be reported in conjunction with D2952, D2953, D2954 or D2957 by the same practitioner.

D3999 **unspecified endodontic procedure, by report**
Used for a procedure that is not adequately described by a code. Describe the procedure.

V. Periodontics

Local anesthesia is usually considered to be part of Periodontal procedures.

Surgical Services (Including Usual Postoperative Care)

Site: A term used to describe a single area, position, or locus. The word "site" is frequently used to indicate an area of soft tissue recession on a single tooth or an osseous defect adjacent to a single tooth; also used to indicate soft tissue defects and/or osseous defects in edentulous tooth positions.

- If two contiguous teeth have areas of soft tissue recession, each tooth is a single site.
- If two contiguous teeth have adjacent but separate osseous defects, each defect is a single site.
- If two contiguous teeth have a communicating interproximal osseous defect, it should be considered a single site.
- All non-communicating osseous defects are single sites.
- All edentulous non-contiguous tooth positions are single sites.
- Up to two contiguous edentulous tooth positions may be considered a single site.

Tooth Bounded Space: A space created by one or more missing teeth that has a tooth on each side.

D4210 **gingivectomy or gingivoplasty – four or more contiguous teeth or tooth bounded spaces per quadrant**
It is performed to eliminate suprabony pockets or to restore normal architecture when gingival enlargements or asymmetrical or unaesthetic topography is evident with normal bony configuration.

D4211 **gingivectomy or gingivoplasty – one to three contiguous teeth or tooth bounded spaces per quadrant**
It is performed to eliminate suprabony pockets or to restore normal architecture when gingival enlargements or asymmetrical or unaesthetic topography is evident with normal bony configuration.

D4212 **gingivectomy or gingivoplasty to allow access for restorative procedure, per tooth**

D4230   **anatomical crown exposure – four or more contiguous teeth or bounded tooth spaces per quadrant**
This procedure is utilized in an otherwise periodontally healthy area to remove enlarged gingival tissue and supporting bone (ostectomy) to provide an anatomically correct gingival relationship.

D4231   **anatomical crown exposure – one to three teeth or bounded tooth spaces per quadrant**
This procedure is utilized in an otherwise periodontally healthy area to remove enlarged gingival tissue and supporting bone (ostectomy) to provide an anatomically correct gingival relationship.

D4240   **gingival flap procedure, including root planing – four or more contiguous teeth or tooth bounded spaces per quadrant**
A soft tissue flap is reflected or resected to allow debridement of the root surface and the removal of granulation tissue. Osseous recontouring is not accomplished in conjunction with this procedure. May include open flap curettage, reverse bevel flap surgery, modified Kirkland flap procedure, and modified Widman surgery. This procedure is performed in the presence of moderate to deep probing depths, loss of attachment, need to maintain esthetics, need for increased access to the root surface and alveolar bone, or to determine the presence of a cracked tooth or fractured root. Other procedures may be required concurrent to D4240 and should be reported separately using their own unique codes.

D4241   **gingival flap procedure, including root planing – one to three contiguous teeth or tooth bounded spaces per quadrant**
A soft tissue flap is reflected or resected to allow debridement of the root surface and the removal of granulation tissue. Osseous recontouring is not accomplished in conjunction with this procedure. May include open flap curettage, reverse bevel flap surgery, modified Kirkland flap procedure, and modified Widman surgery. This procedure is performed in the presence of moderate to deep probing depths, loss of attachment, need to maintain esthetics, need for increased access to the root surface and alveolar bone, or to determine the presence of a cracked tooth or fractured root. Other procedures may be required concurrent to D4241 and should be reported separately using their own unique codes.

D4245 **apically positioned flap**
Procedure is used to preserve keratinized gingiva in conjunction with osseous resection and second stage implant procedure. Procedure may also be used to preserve keratinized/attached gingiva during surgical exposure of labially impacted teeth, and may be used during treatment of peri-implantitis.

D4249 **clinical crown lengthening – hard tissue**
This procedure is employed to allow a restorative procedure on a tooth with little or no tooth structure exposed to the oral cavity. Crown lengthening requires reflection of a full thickness flap and removal of bone, altering the crown to root ratio. It is performed in a healthy periodontal environment, as opposed to osseous surgery, which is performed in the presence of periodontal disease.

D4260 **osseous surgery (including elevation of a full thickness flap and closure) – four or more contiguous teeth or tooth bounded spaces per quadrant**
This procedure modifies the bony support of the teeth by reshaping the alveolar process to achieve a more physiologic form during the surgical procedure. This must include the removal of supporting bone (ostectomy) and/or non-supporting bone (osteoplasty). Other procedures may be required concurrent to D4260 and should be reported using their own unique codes.

D4261 **osseous surgery (including elevation of a full thickness flap and closure) – one to three contiguous teeth or tooth bounded spaces per quadrant**
This procedure modifies the bony support of the teeth by reshaping the alveolar process to achieve a more physiologic form during the surgical procedure. This must include the removal of supporting bone (ostectomy) and/or non-supporting bone (osteoplasty). Other procedures may be required concurrent to D4261 and should be reported using their own unique codes.

D4263 **bone replacement graft – retained natural tooth – first site in quadrant**
This procedure involves the use of grafts to stimulate periodontal regeneration when the disease process has led to a deformity of the bone. This procedure does not include flap entry and closure, wound debridement, osseous contouring, or the placement of biologic materials to aid in osseous tissue regeneration or barrier membranes. Other separate procedures delivered concurrently are documented with their own codes. Not to be reported for an edentulous space or an extraction site.

D4264   **bone replacement graft – retained natural tooth – each additional site in quadrant**
This procedure involves the use of grafts to stimulate periodontal regeneration when the disease process has led to a deformity of the bone. This procedure does not include flap entry and closure, wound debridement, osseous contouring, or the placement of biologic materials to aid in osseous tissue regeneration or barrier membranes. This procedure is performed concurrently with one or more bone replacement grafts to document the number of sites involved.
Not to be reported for an edentulous space or an extraction site.

D4265   **biologic materials to aid in soft and osseous tissue regeneration, per site**
Biologic materials may be used alone or with other regenerative substrates such as bone and barrier membranes, depending upon their formulation and the presentation of the periodontal defect. This procedure does not include surgical entry and closure, wound debridement, osseous contouring, or the placement of graft materials and/or barrier membranes. Other separate procedures may be required concurrent to D4265 and should be reported using their own unique codes.

D4266   **guided tissue regeneration, natural teeth – resorbable barrier, per site**
This procedure does not include flap entry and closure, or, when indicated, wound debridement, osseous contouring, bone replacement grafts, and placement of biologic materials to aid in osseous regeneration. This procedure can be used for periodontal defects around natural teeth.

D4267   **guided tissue regeneration, natural teeth – non-resorbable barrier, per site**
This procedure does not include flap entry and closure, or, when indicated, wound debridement, osseous contouring, bone replacement grafts, and placement of biologic materials to aid in osseous regeneration. This procedure can be used for periodontal defects around natural teeth.

D4286   **removal of non-resorbable barrier**

D4268   **surgical revision procedure, per tooth**
This procedure is to refine the results of a previously provided surgical procedure. This may require a surgical procedure to modify the irregular contours of hard or soft tissue. A mucoperiosteal flap may be elevated to allow access to reshape alveolar bone. The flaps are replaced or repositioned and sutured.

D4270 **pedicle soft tissue graft procedure**
A pedicle flap of gingiva can be raised from an edentulous ridge, adjacent teeth, or from the existing gingiva on the tooth and moved laterally or coronally to replace alveolar mucosa as marginal tissue. The procedure can be used to cover an exposed root or to eliminate a gingival defect if the root is not too prominent in the arch.

D4273 **autogenous connective tissue graft procedure (including donor and recipient surgical sites) first tooth, implant or edentulous tooth position in graft**
There are two surgical sites. The recipient site utilizes a split thickness incision, retaining the overlapping flap of gingiva and/or mucosa. The connective tissue is dissected from a separate donor site leaving an epithelialized flap for closure.

D4283 **autogenous connective tissue graft procedure (including donor and recipient surgical sites) – each additional contiguous tooth, implant or edentulous tooth position in same graft site**
Used in conjunction with D4273.

D4275 **non-autogenous connective tissue graft (including recipient site and donor material) first tooth, implant, or edentulous tooth position in graft**
There is only a recipient surgical site utilizing split thickness incision, retaining the overlaying flap of gingiva and/or mucosa. A donor surgical site is not present.

D4285 **non-autogenous connective tissue graft procedure (including recipient surgical site and donor material) – each additional contiguous tooth, implant or edentulous tooth position in same graft site**
Used in conjunction with D4275.

D4274 **mesial/distal wedge procedure, single tooth (when not performed in conjunction with surgical procedures in the same anatomical area)**
This procedure is performed in an edentulous area adjacent to a tooth, allowing removal of a tissue wedge to gain access for debridement, permit close flap adaptation, and reduce pocket depths.

D4276 **combined connective tissue and pedicle graft, per tooth**
Advanced gingival recession often cannot be corrected with a single procedure. Combined tissue grafting procedures are needed to achieve the desired outcome.

D4277 **free soft tissue graft procedure (including recipient and donor surgical sites) first tooth, implant, or edentulous tooth position in graft**

D4278 **free soft tissue graft procedure (including recipient and donor surgical sites) each additional contiguous tooth, implant, or edentulous tooth position in same graft site**
Used in conjunction with D4277.

Non-Surgical Periodontal Service

D4322 **splint – intra-coronal; natural teeth or prosthetic crowns**
Additional procedure that physically links individual teeth or prosthetic crowns to provide stabilization and additional strength.

D4323 **splint – extra-coronal; natural teeth or prosthetic crowns**
Additional procedure that physically links individual teeth or prosthetic crowns to provide stabilization and additional strength.

D4341 **periodontal scaling and root planing – four or more teeth per quadrant**
This procedure involves instrumentation of the crown and root surfaces of the teeth to remove plaque and calculus from these surfaces. It is indicated for patients with periodontal disease and is therapeutic, not prophylactic, in nature. Root planing is the definitive procedure designed for the removal of cementum and dentin that is rough, and/or permeated by calculus or contaminated with toxins or microorganisms. Some soft tissue removal occurs. This procedure may be used as a definitive treatment in some stages of periodontal disease and/or as a part of pre-surgical procedures in others.

D4342 **periodontal scaling and root planing – one to three teeth per quadrant**
This procedure involves instrumentation of the crown and root surfaces of the teeth to remove plaque and calculus from these surfaces. It is indicated for patients with periodontal disease and is therapeutic, not prophylactic, in nature. Root planing is the definitive procedure designed for the removal of cementum and dentin that is rough, and/or permeated by calculus or contaminated with toxins or microorganisms. Some soft tissue removal occurs. This procedure may be used as a definitive treatment in some stages of periodontal disease and/or as a part of pre-surgical procedures in others.

D4346   **scaling in presence of generalized moderate or severe gingival inflammation – full mouth, after oral evaluation**
The removal of plaque, calculus and stains from supra- and sub-gingival tooth surfaces when there is generalized moderate or severe gingival inflammation in the absence of periodontitis. It is indicated for patients who have swollen, inflamed gingiva, generalized suprabony pockets, and moderate to severe bleeding on probing. Should not be reported in conjunction with prophylaxis, scaling and root planing, or debridement procedures.

D4355   **full mouth debridement to enable a comprehensive periodontal evaluation and diagnosis on a subsequent visit**

D4381   **localized delivery of antimicrobial agents via a controlled release vehicle into diseased crevicular tissue, per tooth**
FDA approved subgingival delivery devices containing antimicrobial medication(s) are inserted into periodontal pockets to suppress the pathogenic microbiota. These devices slowly release the pharmacological agents so they can remain at the intended site of action in a therapeutic concentration for a sufficient length of time.

Other Periodontal Services

D4910   **periodontal maintenance**
This procedure is instituted following periodontal therapy and continues at varying intervals, determined by the clinical evaluation of the dentist, for the life of the dentition or any implant replacements. It includes removal of the bacterial plaque and calculus from supragingival and subgingival regions, site specific scaling and root planing where indicated, and polishing the teeth. If new or recurring periodontal disease appears, additional diagnostic and treatment procedures must be considered.

D4920   **unscheduled dressing change (by someone other than treating dentist or their staff)**

D4921   **gingival irrigation with a medicinal agent – per quadrant**

D4999   **unspecified periodontal procedure, by report**
Use for a procedure that is not adequately described by a code. Describe the procedure.

Section 1: Code on Dental Procedures and Nomenclature

VI. Prosthodontics, removable

Local anesthesia is usually considered to be part of Removable Prosthodontic procedures.

Complete Dentures (Including Routine Post-Delivery Care)

D5110   **complete denture – maxillary**

D5120   **complete denture – mandibular**

D5130   **immediate denture – maxillary**
Includes limited follow-up care only; does not include future rebasing/relining procedure(s).

D5140   **immediate denture – mandibular**
Includes limited follow-up care only; does not include future rebasing/relining procedure(s).

Partial Dentures (Including Routine Post-Delivery Care)

D5211   **maxillary partial denture – resin base (including retentive/clasping materials, rests, and teeth)**

D5212   **mandibular partial denture – resin base (including retentive/clasping materials, rests, and teeth)**

D5213   **maxillary partial denture – cast metal framework with resin denture bases (including retentive/clasping materials, rests and teeth)**

D5214   **mandibular partial denture – cast metal framework with resin denture bases (including retentive/clasping materials, rests and teeth)**

D5225   **maxillary partial denture – flexible base (including retentive/clasping materials, rests, and teeth)**

D5226   **mandibular partial denture – flexible base (including retentive/clasping materials, rests, and teeth)**

D5221   **immediate maxillary partial denture – resin base (including retentive/clasping materials, rests and teeth)**
Includes limited follow-up care only; does not include future rebasing/relining procedure(s).

D5222 **immediate mandibular partial denture – resin base (including retentive/clasping materials, rests and teeth)**
Includes limited follow-up care only; does not include future rebasing/relining procedure(s).

D5223 **immediate maxillary partial denture – cast metal framework with resin denture bases (including retentive/clasping materials, rests and teeth)**
Includes limited follow-up care only; does not include future rebasing/relining procedure(s).

D5224 **immediate mandibular partial denture – cast metal framework with resin denture bases (including retentive/clasping materials, rests and teeth)**
Includes limited follow-up care only; does not include future rebasing/relining procedure(s).

D5227 **immediate maxillary partial denture – flexible base (including any clasps, rests and teeth)**

D5228 **immediate mandibular partial denture – flexible base (including any clasps, rests and teeth)**

D5282 **removable unilateral partial denture – one piece cast metal (including retentive/clasping materials, rests, and teeth), maxillary**

D5283 **removable unilateral partial denture – one piece cast metal (including retentive/clasping materials, rests, and teeth), mandibular**

D5284 **removable unilateral partial denture – one piece flexible base (including retentive/clasping materials, rests, and teeth) – per quadrant**

D5286 **removable unilateral partial denture – one piece resin (including retentive/clasping materials, rests, and teeth) – per quadrant**

Adjustments to Dentures

D5410 **adjust complete denture – maxillary**

D5411 **adjust complete denture – mandibular**

D5421 **adjust partial denture – maxillary**

D5422 **adjust partial denture – mandibular**

Repairs to Complete Dentures

D5511	repair broken complete denture base, mandibular
D5512	repair broken complete denture base, maxillary
D5520	replace missing or broken teeth – complete denture (each tooth)

Repairs to Partial Dentures

D5611	repair resin partial denture base, mandibular
D5612	repair resin partial denture base, maxillary
D5621	repair cast partial framework, mandibular
D5622	repair cast partial framework, maxillary
D5630	repair or replace broken retentive/clasping materials – per tooth
D5640	replace broken teeth – per tooth
D5650	add tooth to existing partial denture
D5660	add clasp to existing partial denture – per tooth
D5670	replace all teeth and acrylic on cast metal framework (maxillary)
D5671	replace all teeth and acrylic on cast metal framework (mandibular)

Denture Rebase Procedures

Rebase – process of refitting a denture by replacing the base material.

D5710	rebase complete maxillary denture
D5711	rebase complete mandibular denture
D5720	rebase maxillary partial denture
D5721	rebase mandibular partial denture
D5725	rebase hybrid prosthesis
	Replacing the base material connected to the framework.

Denture Reline Procedures

Reline is the process of resurfacing the tissue side of a denture with new base material.

D5730   **reline complete maxillary denture (direct)**

D5731   **reline complete mandibular denture (direct)**

D5740   **reline maxillary partial denture (direct)**

D5741   **reline mandibular partial denture (direct)**

D5750   **reline complete maxillary denture (indirect)**

D5751   **reline complete mandibular denture (indirect)**

D5760   **reline maxillary partial denture (indirect)**

D5761   **reline mandibular partial denture (indirect)**

Interim Prosthesis

A prosthesis designed for use over a limited period of time, after which it is to be replaced by a definitive restoration.

D5810   **interim complete denture (maxillary)**

D5811   **interim complete denture (mandibular)**

D5820   **interim partial denture (including retentive/clasping materials, rests, and teeth), maxillary**

D5821   **interim partial denture (including retentive/clasping materials, rests, and teeth), mandibular**

Other Removable Prosthetic Services

D5765   **soft liner for complete or partial removable denture – indirect**
A discrete procedure provided when the dentist determines placement of the soft liner is clinically indicated.

D5850   **tissue conditioning, maxillary**
Treatment reline using materials designed to heal unhealthy ridges prior to more definitive final restoration.

D5851   **tissue conditioning, mandibular**
Treatment reline using materials designed to heal unhealthy ridges prior to more definitive final restoration.

D5862 **precision attachment, by report**
Each pair of components is one precision attachment. Describe the type of attachment used.

D5863 **overdenture – complete maxillary**

D5864 **overdenture – partial maxillary**

D5865 **overdenture – complete mandibular**

D5866 **overdenture – partial mandibular**

D5867 **replacement of replaceable part of semi-precision or precision attachment, per attachment**

D5875 **modification of removable prosthesis following implant surgery**
Attachment assemblies are reported using separate codes.

▲ **D5876** **add metal substructure to acrylic full denture (per arch)**
Use of metal substructure in removable complete dentures without a framework.

D5899 **unspecified removable prosthodontic procedure, by report**
Use for a procedure that is not adequately described by a code. Describe the procedure.

VII. Maxillofacial Prosthetics

D5992 **adjust maxillofacial prosthetic appliance, by report**

D5993 **maintenance and cleaning of a maxillofacial prosthesis (extra- or intra-oral) other than required adjustments, by report**

D5914 **auricular prosthesis**

Synonymous terminology: artificial ear, ear prosthesis.

A removable prosthesis, which artificially restores part or all of the natural ear. Usually, replacement prostheses can be made from the original mold if tissue bed changes have not occurred. Creation of an auricular prosthesis requires fabrication of a mold, from which additional prostheses usually can be made, as needed later (auricular prosthesis, replacement).

D5927 **auricular prosthesis, replacement**

Synonymous terminology: replacement ear.

An artificial ear produced from a previously made mold. A replacement prosthesis does not require fabrication of a new mold. Generally, several prostheses can be made from the same mold assuming no changes occur in the tissue bed due to surgery or age related topographical variations.

D5987 **commissure splint**

Synonymous terminology: lip splint.

A device placed between the lips, which assists in achieving increased opening between the lips. Use of such devices enhances opening where surgical, chemical or electrical alterations of the lips has resulted in severe restriction or contractures.

D5924 **cranial prosthesis**

Synonymous terminology: Skull plate, cranioplasty prosthesis, cranial implant.

A biocompatible, permanently implanted replacement of a portion of the skull bones; an artificial replacement for a portion of the skull bone.

D5925 **facial augmentation implant prosthesis**

Synonymous terminology: facial implant.

An implantable biocompatible material generally onlayed upon an existing bony area beneath the skin tissue to fill in or collectively raise portions of the overlaying facial skin tissues to create acceptable contours.

Although some forms of pre-made surgical implants are commercially available, the facial augmentation is usually custom made for surgical implantation for each individual patient due to the irregular or extensive nature of the facial deficit.

Section 1: Code on Dental Procedures and Nomenclature

D5912 **facial moulage (complete)**
Synonymous terminology: facial impression, face mask impression.

A complete facial moulage impression is a procedure used to record the soft tissue contours of the whole face. The impression is utilized to create a facial moulage and generally is not reusable.

D5911 **facial moulage (sectional)**
A sectional facial moulage impression is a procedure used to record the soft tissue contours of a portion of the face. Occasionally several separate sectional impressions are made, and then reassembled to provide a full facial contour cast. The impression is utilized to create a partial facial moulage and generally is not reusable.

D5919 **facial prosthesis**
Synonymous terminology: prosthetic dressing.

A removable prosthesis, which artificially replaces a portion of the face, lost due to surgery, trauma or congenital absence.

Flexion of natural tissues may preclude adaptation and movement of the prosthesis to match the adjacent skin. Salivary leakage, when communicating with the oral cavity, adversely affects retention.

D5929 **facial prosthesis, replacement**
A replacement facial prosthesis made from the original mold.

A replacement prosthesis does not require fabrication of a new mold. Generally, several prostheses can be made from the same mold assuming no changes occur in the tissue bed due to further surgery or age related topographical variations.

D5951 **feeding aid**
Synonymous terminology: feeding prosthesis.

A prosthesis, which maintains the right and left maxillary segments of an infant cleft palate patient in their proper orientation until surgery is performed to repair the cleft. It closes the oral–nasal cavity defect, thus enhancing sucking and swallowing.

Used on an interim basis, this prosthesis achieves separation of the oral and nasal cavities in infants born with wide clefts necessitating delayed closure. It is eliminated if surgical closure can be effected or, alternatively, with eruption of the deciduous dentition a pediatric speech aid may be made to facilitate closure of the defect.

D5934 **mandibular resection prosthesis with guide flange**
Synonymous terminology: resection device, resection appliance.

A prosthesis which guides the remaining portion of the mandible, left after a partial resection, into a more normal relationship with the maxilla. This allows for some tooth-to-tooth or an improved tooth contact. It may also artificially replace missing teeth and thereby increase masticatory efficiency.

D5935 **mandibular resection prosthesis without guide flange**
A prosthesis which helps guide the partially resected mandible to a more normal relation with the maxilla allowing for increased tooth contact. It does not have a flange or ramp, however, to assist in directional closure. It may replace missing teeth and thereby increase masticatory efficiency.

Dentists who treat mandibulectomy patients may prefer to replace some, all or none of the teeth in the defect area. Frequently, the defect's margins preclude even partial replacement. Use of a guide (a mandibular resection prosthesis with a guide flange) may not be possible due to anatomical limitations or poor patient tolerance. Ramps, extended occlusal arrangements and irregular occlusal positioning relative to the denture foundation frequently preclude stability of the prostheses, and thus some prostheses are poorly tolerated under such adverse circumstances.

D5913 **nasal prosthesis**
Synonymous terminology: artificial nose.

A removable prosthesis attached to the skin, which artificially restores part or all of the nose. Fabrication of a nasal prosthesis requires creation of an original mold. Additional prostheses usually can be made from the same mold, and assuming no further tissue changes occur, the same mold can be utilized for extended periods of time.

When a new prosthesis is made from the existing mold, this procedure is termed a nasal prosthesis replacement.

D5926 **nasal prosthesis, replacement**
Synonymous terminology: replacement nose.

An artificial nose produced from a previously made mold. A replacement prosthesis does not require fabrication of a new mold. Generally, several prostheses can be made from the same mold assuming no changes occur in the tissue bed due to surgery or age related topographical variations.

D5922   nasal septal prosthesis

Synonymous terminology: Septal plug, septal button.

Removable prosthesis to occlude (obturate) a hole within the nasal septal wall. Adverse chemical degradation in this moist environment may require frequent replacement. Silicone prostheses are occasionally subject to fungal invasion.

D5932   obturator prosthesis, definitive

Synonymous terminology: obturator.

A prosthesis, which artificially replaces part or all of the maxilla and associated teeth, lost due to surgery, trauma or congenital defects.

A definitive obturator is made when it is deemed that further tissue changes or recurrence of tumor are unlikely and a more permanent prosthetic rehabilitation can be achieved; it is intended for long-term use.

D5936   obturator prosthesis, interim

Synonymous terminology: immediate postoperative obturator.

A prosthesis which is made following completion of the initial healing after a surgical resection of a portion or all of one or both the maxillae; frequently many or all teeth in the defect area are replaced by this prosthesis. This prosthesis replaces the surgical obturator, which is usually inserted at, or immediately following the resection.

Generally, an interim obturator is made to facilitate closure of the resultant defect after initial healing has been completed. Unlike the surgical obturator, which usually is made prior to surgery and frequently revised in the operating room during surgery, the interim obturator is made when the defect margins are clearly defined and further surgical revisions are not planned. It is a provisional prosthesis, which may replace some or all lost teeth, and other lost bone and soft tissue structures. Also, it frequently must be revised (termed an obturator prosthesis modification) during subsequent dental procedures (e.g., restorations, gingival surgery) as well as to compensate for further tissue shrinkage before a definitive obturator prosthesis is made.

D5933   obturator prosthesis, modification

Synonymous terminology: adjustment, denture adjustment, temporary or office reline.

Revision or alteration of an existing obturator (surgical, interim, or definitive); possible modifications include relief of the denture base due to tissue compression, augmentation of the seal or peripheral areas to effect adequate sealing or separation between the nasal and oral cavities.

D5931 **obturator prosthesis, surgical**

Synonymous terminology: Obturator, surgical stayplate, immediate temporary obturator.

A temporary prosthesis inserted during or immediately following surgical or traumatic loss of a portion or all of one or both maxillary bones and contiguous alveolar structures (e.g., gingival tissue, teeth).

Frequent revisions of surgical obturators are necessary during the ensuing healing phase (approximately six months). Some dentists prefer to replace many or all teeth removed by the surgical procedure in the surgical obturator, while others do not replace any teeth. Further surgical revisions may require fabrication of another surgical obturator (e.g., an initially planned small defect may be revised and greatly enlarged after the final pathology report indicates margins are not free of tumor).

D5916 **ocular prosthesis**

Synonymous terminology: artificial eye, glass eye.

A prosthesis, which artificially replaces an eye missing as a result of trauma, surgery or congenital absence. The prosthesis does not replace missing eyelids or adjacent skin, mucosa or muscle.

Ocular prostheses require semiannual or annual cleaning and polishing. Also, occasional revisions to re-adapt the prosthesis to the tissue bed may be necessary. Glass eyes are rarely made and cannot be re-adapted.

D5923 **ocular prosthesis, interim**

Synonymous terminology: Eye shell, shell, ocular conformer, conformer.

A temporary replacement generally made of clear acrylic resin for an eye lost due to surgery or trauma. No attempt is made to re-establish esthetics. Fabrication of an interim ocular prosthesis generally implies subsequent fabrication of an aesthetic ocular prosthesis.

D5915 **orbital prosthesis**

A prosthesis, which artificially restores the eye, eyelids, and adjacent hard and soft tissue, lost as a result of trauma or surgery.

Fabrication of an orbital prosthesis requires creation of an original mold. Additional prostheses usually can be made from the same mold, and assuming no further tissue changes occur, the same mold can be utilized for extended periods of time.

When a new prosthesis is made from the existing mold, this procedure is termed an orbital prosthesis replacement.

D5928 **orbital prosthesis, replacement**
A replacement for a previously made orbital prosthesis. A replacement prosthesis does not require fabrication of a new mold. Generally, several prostheses can be made from the same mold assuming no changes occur in the tissue bed due to surgery or age related topographical variations.

D5954 **palatal augmentation prosthesis**
Synonymous terminology: superimposed prosthesis, maxillary glossectomy prosthesis, maxillary speech prosthesis, palatal drop prosthesis.

A removable prosthesis which alters the hard and/or soft palate's topographical form adjacent to the tongue.

D5955 **palatal lift prosthesis, definitive**
A prosthesis which elevates the soft palate superiorly and aids in restoration of soft palate functions which may be lost due to an acquired, congenital or developmental defect.

A definitive palatal lift is usually made for patients whose experience with an interim palatal lift has been successful, especially if surgical alterations are deemed unwarranted.

D5958 **palatal lift prosthesis, interim**
Synonymous terminology: diagnostic palatal lift.

A prosthesis which elevates and assists in restoring soft palate function which may be lost due to clefting, surgery, trauma or unknown paralysis. It is intended for interim use to determine its usefulness in achieving palatalpharyngeal competency or enhance swallowing reflexes.

This prosthesis is intended for interim use as a diagnostic aid to assess the level of possible improvement in speech intelligibility. Some clinicians believe use of a palatal lift on an interim basis may stimulate an otherwise flaccid soft palate to increase functional activity, subsequently lessening its need.

D5959 **palatal lift prosthesis, modification**
Synonymous terminology: revision of lift, adjustment.

Alterations in the adaptation, contour, form or function of an existing palatal lift necessitated due to tissue impingement, lack of function, poor clasp adaptation or the like.

D5985 **radiation cone locator**
Synonymous terminology: docking device, cone locator.

A prosthesis utilized to direct and reduplicate the path of radiation to an oral tumor during a split course of irradiation.

D5984 **radiation shield**

Synonymous terminology: radiation stent, tongue protector, lead shield.

An intraoral prosthesis designed to shield adjacent tissues from radiation during orthovoltage treatment of malignant lesions of the head and neck region.

D5953 **speech aid prosthesis, adult**

Synonymous terminology: prosthetic speech appliance, speech aid, speech bulb.

A definitive prosthesis, which can improve speech in adult cleft palate patients either by obturating (sealing off) a palatal cleft or fistula, or occasionally by assisting an incompetent soft palate. Both mechanisms are necessary to achieve velopharyngeal competency.

Generally, this prosthesis is fabricated when no further growth is anticipated and the objective is to achieve long-term use. Hence, more precise materials and techniques are utilized. Occasionally such procedures are accomplished in conjunction with precision attachments in crown work undertaken on some or all maxillary teeth to achieve improved aesthetics.

D5960 **speech aid prosthesis, modification**

Synonymous terminology: adjustment, repair, revision.

Any revision of a pediatric or adult speech aid not necessitating its replacement.

Frequently, revisions of the obturating section of any speech aid are required to facilitate enhanced speech intelligibility. Such revisions or repairs do not require complete remaking of the prosthesis, thus extending its longevity.

D5952 **speech aid prosthesis, pediatric**

Synonymous terminology: nasopharyngeal obturator, speech appliance, obturator, cleft palate appliance, prosthetic speech aid, speech bulb.

A temporary or interim prosthesis used to close a defect in the hard and/or soft palate. It may replace tissue lost due to developmental or surgical alterations. It is necessary for the production of intelligible speech.

Normal lateral growth of the palatal bones necessitates occasional replacement of this prosthesis. Intermittent revisions of the obturator section can assist in maintenance of palatalpharyngeal closure (termed a speech aid prosthesis modification). Frequently, such prostheses are not fabricated before the deciduous dentition is fully erupted since clasp retention is often essential.

Section 1: Code on Dental Procedures and Nomenclature

D5988   surgical splint

Synonymous terminology: Gunning splint, modified Gunning splint, labiolingual splint, fenestrated splint, Kingsley splint, cast metal splint.

Splints are designed to utilize existing teeth and/or alveolar processes as points of anchorage to assist in stabilization and immobilization of broken bones during healing. They are used to re-establish, as much as possible, normal occlusal relationships during the process of immobilization. Frequently, existing prostheses (e.g., a patient's complete dentures) can be modified to serve as surgical splints. Frequently, surgical splints have arch bars added to facilitate intermaxillary fixation. Rubber elastics may be used to assist in this process. Circummandibular eyelet hooks can be utilized for enhanced stabilization with wiring to adjacent bone.

D5982   surgical stent

Synonymous terminology: periodontal stent, skin graft stent, columellar stent.

Stents are utilized to apply pressure to soft tissues to facilitate healing and prevent cicatrization or collapse.

A surgical stent may be required in surgical and post-surgical revisions to achieve close approximation of tissues. Usually such materials as temporary or interim soft denture liners, gutta percha, or dental modeling impression compound may be used.

D5937   trismus appliance (not for TMD treatment)

Synonymous terminology: occlusal device for mandibular trismus, dynamic bite opener.

A prosthesis, which assists the patient in increasing their oral aperture width in order to eat as well as maintain oral hygiene.

Several versions and designs are possible, all intending to ease the severe lack of oral opening experienced by many patients immediately following extensive intraoral surgical procedures.

Carriers

D5986   fluoride gel carrier

Synonymous terminology: fluoride applicator.

A prosthesis, which covers the teeth in either dental arch and is used to apply topical fluoride in close proximity to tooth enamel and dentin for several minutes daily.

D5995 **periodontal medicament carrier with peripheral seal – laboratory processed – maxillary**

A custom fabricated, laboratory processed carrier for the maxillary arch that covers the teeth and alveolar mucosa. Used as a vehicle to deliver prescribed medicaments for sustained contact with the gingiva, alveolar mucosa, and into the periodontal sulcus or pocket.

D5996 **periodontal medicament carrier with peripheral seal – laboratory processed – mandibular**

A custom fabricated, laboratory processed carrier for the mandibular arch that covers the teeth and alveolar mucosa. Used as a vehicle to deliver prescribed medicaments for sustained contact with the gingiva, alveolar mucosa, and into the periodontal sulcus or pocket.

D5983 **radiation carrier**

Synonymous terminology: radiotherapy prosthesis, carrier prosthesis, radiation applicator, radium carrier, intracavity carrier, intracavity applicator.

A device used to administer radiation to confined areas by means of capsules, beads or needles of radiation emitting materials such as radium or cesium. Its function is to hold the radiation source securely in the same location during the entire period of treatment.

Radiation oncologists occasionally request these devices to achieve close approximation and controlled application of radiation to a tumor deemed amiable to eradication.

D5991 **vesiculobullous disease medicament carrier**

A custom fabricated carrier that covers the teeth and alveolar mucosa, or alveolar mucosa alone, and is used to deliver prescription medicaments for treatment of immunologically mediated vesiculobullous diseases.

D5999 **unspecified maxillofacial prosthesis, by report**

Used for a procedure that is not adequately described by a code. Describe the procedure.

VIII. Implant Services

Local anesthesia is usually considered to be part of Implant Services procedures.

Pre-Surgical Services

D6190 **radiographic/surgical implant index, by report**
An appliance, designed to relate osteotomy or fixture position to existing anatomic structures, to be utilized during radiographic exposure for treatment planning and/or during osteotomy creation for fixture installation.

Surgical Services

Report surgical implant procedure using codes in this section.

D6010 **surgical placement of implant body: endosteal implant**

D6011 **surgical access to an implant body (second stage implant surgery)**
This procedure, also known as second stage implant surgery, involves removal of tissue that covers the implant body so that a fixture of any type can be placed, or an existing fixture be replaced with another. Examples of fixtures include but are not limited to healing caps, abutments shaped to help contour the gingival margins or the final restorative prosthesis.

D6012 **surgical placement of interim implant body for transitional prosthesis: endosteal implant**

D6013 **surgical placement of mini implant**

D6040 **surgical placement: eposteal implant**
An eposteal (subperiosteal) framework of a biocompatible material designed and fabricated to fit on the surface of the bone of the mandible or maxilla with permucosal extensions which provide support and attachment of a prosthesis. This may be a complete arch or unilateral appliance. Eposteal implants rest upon the bone and under the periosteum.

D6050 **surgical placement: transosteal implant**
A transosteal (transosseous) biocompatible device with threaded posts penetrating both the superior and inferior cortical bone plates of the mandibular symphysis and exiting through the permucosa providing support and attachment for a dental prosthesis. Transosteal implants are placed completely through the bone and into the oral cavity from extraoral or intraoral.

D6100 **surgical removal of implant body**

D6101 **debridement of a peri-implant defect or defects surrounding a single implant, and surface cleaning of the exposed implant surfaces, including flap entry and closure**

D6102 **debridement and osseous contouring of a peri-implant defect or defects surrounding a single implant and includes surface cleaning of the exposed implant surfaces, including flap entry and closure**

D6103 **bone graft for repair of peri-implant defect – does not include flap entry and closure**
Placement of a barrier membrane or biologic materials to aid in osseous regeneration, are reported separately.

D6104 **bone graft at time of implant placement**
Placement of a barrier membrane, or biologic materials to aid in osseous regeneration are reported separately.

D6105 **removal of implant body not requiring bone removal or flap elevation**

D6106 **guided tissue regeneration – resorbable barrier, per implant**
This procedure does not include flap entry and closure, or, when indicated, wound debridement, osseous contouring, bone replacement grafts, and placement of biologic materials to aid in osseous regeneration. This procedure is used for peri-implant defects and during implant placement.

D6107 **guided tissue regeneration – non-resorbable barrier, per implant**
This procedure does not include flap entry and closure, or, when indicated, wound debridement, osseous contouring, bone replacement grafts, and placement of biologic materials to aid in osseous regeneration. This procedure is used for peri-implant defects and during implant placement.

Implant Supported Prosthetics

Supporting Structures

D6055 **connecting bar – implant supported or abutment supported**
Utilized to stabilize and anchor a prosthesis.

D6056 **prefabricated abutment – includes modification and placement**
Modification of a prefabricated abutment may be necessary.

D6057 **custom fabricated abutment – includes placement**
Created by a laboratory process, specific for an individual application.

D6051 **interim implant abutment placement**
A healing cap is not an interim abutment.

Section 1: Code on Dental Procedures and Nomenclature

D6191   **semi-precision abutment – placement**
This procedure is the initial placement, or replacement, of a semi-precision abutment on the implant body.

D6192   **semi-precision attachment – placement**
This procedure involves the luting of the initial, or replacement, semi-precision attachment to the removable prosthesis.

Implant/Abutment Supported Removable Dentures

D6110   **implant/abutment supported removable denture for edentulous arch – maxillary**

D6111   **implant/abutment supported removable denture for edentulous arch – mandibular**

D6112   **implant/abutment supported removable denture for partially edentulous arch – maxillary**

D6113   **implant/abutment supported removable denture for partially edentulous arch – mandibular**

Implant/Abutment Supported Fixed Dentures (Hybrid Prosthesis)

D6114   **implant/abutment supported fixed denture for edentulous arch – maxillary**

D6115   **implant/abutment supported fixed denture for edentulous arch – mandibular**

D6116   **implant/abutment supported fixed denture for partially edentulous arch – maxillary**

D6117   **implant/abutment supported fixed denture for partially edentulous arch – mandibular**

D6118   **implant/abutment supported interim fixed denture for edentulous arch – mandibular**
Used when a period of healing is necessary prior to fabrication and placement of a permanent prosthetic.

D6119   **implant/abutment supported interim fixed denture for edentulous arch – maxillary**
Used when a period of healing is necessary prior to fabrication and placement of a permanent prosthetic.

Single Crowns, Abutment Supported

D6058   abutment supported porcelain/ceramic crown
A single crown restoration that is retained, supported and stabilized by an abutment on an implant.

D6059   abutment supported porcelain fused to metal crown (high noble metal)
A single metal-ceramic crown restoration that is retained, supported and stabilized by an abutment on an implant.

D6060   abutment supported porcelain fused to metal crown (predominantly base metal)
A single metal-ceramic crown restoration that is retained, supported and stabilized by an abutment on an implant.

D6061   abutment supported porcelain fused to metal crown (noble metal)
A single metal-ceramic crown restoration that is retained, supported and stabilized by an abutment on an implant.

D6097   abutment supported crown – porcelain fused to titanium or titanium alloys
A single metal-ceramic crown restoration that is retained, supported, and stabilized by an abutment on an implant.

D6062   abutment supported cast metal crown (high noble metal)
A single cast metal crown restoration that is retained, supported and stabilized by an abutment on an implant.

D6063   abutment supported cast metal crown (predominantly base metal)
A single cast metal crown restoration that is retained, supported and stabilized by an abutment on an implant.

D6064   abutment supported cast metal crown (noble metal)
A single cast metal crown restoration that is retained, supported and stabilized by an abutment on an implant.

D6094   abutment supported crown – titanium and titanium alloys
A single crown restoration that is retained, supported and stabilized by an abutment on an implant.

Section 1: Code on Dental Procedures and Nomenclature

Single Crowns, Implant Supported

D6065   **implant supported porcelain/ceramic crown**
A single crown restoration that is retained, supported and stabilized by an implant.

D6066   **implant supported crown – porcelain fused to high noble alloys**
A single metal-ceramic crown restoration that is retained, supported and stabilized by an implant.

D6082   **implant supported crown – porcelain fused to predominantly base alloys**
A single metal-ceramic crown restoration that is retained, supported and stabilized by an implant.

D6083   **implant supported crown – porcelain fused to noble alloys**
A single metal-ceramic crown restoration that is retained, supported and stabilized by an implant.

D6084   **implant supported crown – porcelain fused to titanium or titanium alloys**
A single metal-ceramic crown restoration that is retained, supported and stabilized by an implant.

D6067   **implant supported crown – high noble alloys**
A single metal crown restoration that is retained, supported and stabilized by an implant.

D6086   **implant supported crown – predominantly base alloys**
A single metal crown restoration that is retained, supported and stabilized by an implant.

D6087   **implant supported crown – noble alloys**
A single metal crown restoration that is retained, supported and stabilized by an implant.

D6088   **implant supported crown – titanium and titanium alloys**
A single metal crown restoration that is retained, supported and stabilized by an implant.

Fixed Partial Denture (FPD) Retainer, Abutment Supported

D6068   **abutment supported retainer for porcelain/ceramic FPD**
A ceramic retainer for a fixed partial denture that gains retention, support and stability from an abutment on an implant.

D6069   **abutment supported retainer for porcelain fused to metal FPD (high noble metal)**
A metal-ceramic retainer for a fixed partial denture that gains retention, support and stability from an abutment on an implant.

D6070   **abutment supported retainer for porcelain fused to metal FPD (predominantly base metal)**
A metal-ceramic retainer for a fixed partial denture that gains retention, support and stability from an abutment on an implant.

D6071   **abutment supported retainer for porcelain fused to metal FPD (noble metal)**
A metal-ceramic retainer for a fixed partial denture that gains retention, support and stability from an abutment on an implant.

D6195   **abutment supported retainer – porcelain fused to titanium and titanium alloys**
A metal-ceramic retainer for a fixed partial denture that gains retention, support, and stability from an abutment on an implant.

D6072   **abutment supported retainer for cast metal FPD (high noble metal)**
A cast metal retainer for a fixed partial denture that gains retention, support and stability from an abutment on an implant.

D6073   **abutment supported retainer for cast metal FPD (predominantly base metal)**
A cast metal retainer for a fixed partial denture that gains retention, support and stability from an abutment on an implant.

D6074   **abutment supported retainer for cast metal FPD (noble metal)**
A cast metal retainer for a fixed partial denture that gains retention, support and stability from an abutment on an implant.

D6194   **abutment supported retainer crown for FPD – titanium and titanium alloys**
A retainer for a fixed partial denture that gains retention, support and stability from an abutment on an implant.

Fixed Partial Denture (FPD) Retainer, Implant Supported

D6075   **implant supported retainer for ceramic FPD**
A ceramic retainer for a fixed partial denture that gains retention, support and stability from an implant.

D6076   **implant supported retainer for FPD – porcelain fused to high noble alloys**
A metal-ceramic retainer for a fixed partial denture that gains retention, support and stability from an implant.

D6098   **implant supported retainer – porcelain fused to predominantly base alloys**
A metal-ceramic retainer for a fixed partial denture that gains retention, support, and stability from an implant.

D6099   **implant supported retainer for FPD – porcelain fused to noble alloys**
A metal-ceramic retainer for a fixed partial denture that gains retention, support, and stability from an implant.

D6120   **implant supported retainer – porcelain fused to titanium and titanium alloys**
A metal-ceramic retainer for a fixed partial denture that gains retention, support, and stability from an implant.

D6077   **implant supported retainer for metal FPD – high noble alloys**
A metal retainer for a fixed partial denture that gains retention, support and stability from an implant.

D6121   **implant supported retainer for metal FPD – predominantly base alloys**
A metal retainer for a fixed partial denture that gains retention, support, and stability from an implant.

D6122   **implant supported retainer for metal FPD – noble alloys**
A metal retainer for a fixed partial denture that gains retention, support, and stability from an implant.

D6123   **implant supported retainer for metal FPD – titanium and titanium alloys**
A metal retainer for a fixed partial denture that gains retention, support, and stability from an implant.

Other Implant Services

D6080 **implant maintenance procedures when prostheses are removed and reinserted, including cleansing of prostheses and abutments**
This procedure includes active debriding of the implant(s) and examination of all aspects of the implant system(s), including the occlusion and stability of the superstructure. The patient is also instructed in thorough daily cleansing of the implant(s). This is not a per implant code, and is indicated for implant supported fixed prostheses.

D6081 **scaling and debridement in the presence of inflammation or mucositis of a single implant, including cleaning of the implant surfaces, without flap entry and closure**
This procedure is not performed in conjunction with D1110, D4910, or D4346.

D6085 **interim implant crown**
Placed when a period of healing is necessary prior to fabrication and placement of the definitive prosthesis.

D6090 **repair implant supported prosthesis, by report**
This procedure involves the repair or replacement of any part of the implant supported prosthesis.

D6091 **replacement of replaceable part of semi-precision or precision attachment of implant/abutment supported prosthesis, per attachment**

D6092 **re-cement or re-bond implant/abutment supported crown**

D6093 **re-cement or re-bond implant/abutment supported fixed partial denture**

D6095 **repair implant abutment, by report**
This procedure involves the repair or replacement of any part of the implant abutment.

• **D6089** **accessing and retorquing loose implant screw - per screw**

D6096 **remove broken implant retaining screw**

D6197 **replacement of restorative material used to close an access opening of a screw-retained implant supported prosthesis, per implant**

Section 1: Code on Dental Procedures and Nomenclature

D6198   **remove interim implant component**
Removal of implant component (e.g., interim abutment; provisional implant crown) originally placed for a specific clinical purpose and period of time determined by the dentist.

D6199   **unspecified implant procedure, by report**
Use for a procedure that is not adequately described by a code. Describe the procedure.

IX. Prosthodontics, fixed

Local anesthesia is usually considered to be part of Fixed Prosthodontic procedures.

The term "fixed partial denture" or FPD is synonymous with fixed bridge or bridgework.

Each retainer and each pontic constitutes a unit in a fixed partial denture.

Fixed partial denture prosthetic procedures include routine temporary prosthetics. When indicated, interim or provisional codes should be reported separately.

Fixed Partial Denture Pontics

D6205 **pontic – indirect resin based composite**
Not to be used as a temporary or provisional prosthesis.

D6210 **pontic – cast high noble metal**

D6211 **pontic – cast predominantly base metal**

D6212 **pontic – cast noble metal**

D6214 **pontic – titanium and titanium alloys**

D6240 **pontic – porcelain fused to high noble metal**

D6241 **pontic – porcelain fused to predominantly base metal**

D6242 **pontic – porcelain fused to noble metal**

D6243 **pontic – porcelain fused to titanium and titanium alloys**

D6245 **pontic – porcelain/ceramic**

D6250 **pontic – resin with high noble metal**

D6251 **pontic – resin with predominantly base metal**

D6252 **pontic – resin with noble metal**

D6253 **interim pontic – further treatment or completion of diagnosis necessary prior to final impression**
Not to be used as a temporary pontic for a routine prosthetic restoration.

Section 1: Code on Dental Procedures and Nomenclature

Fixed Partial Denture Retainers – Inlays/Onlays

D6545	retainer – cast metal for resin bonded fixed prosthesis
D6548	retainer – porcelain/ceramic for resin bonded fixed prosthesis
D6549	resin retainer – for resin bonded fixed prosthesis
D6600	retainer inlay – porcelain/ceramic, two surfaces
D6601	retainer inlay – porcelain/ceramic, three or more surfaces
D6602	retainer inlay – cast high noble metal, two surfaces
D6603	retainer inlay – cast high noble metal, three or more surfaces
D6604	retainer inlay – cast predominantly base metal, two surfaces
D6605	retainer inlay – cast predominantly base metal, three or more surfaces
D6606	retainer inlay – cast noble metal, two surfaces
D6607	retainer inlay – cast noble metal, three or more surfaces
D6624	retainer inlay – titanium
D6608	retainer onlay – porcelain/ceramic, two surfaces
D6609	retainer onlay – porcelain/ceramic, three or more surfaces
D6610	retainer onlay – cast high noble metal, two surfaces
D6611	retainer onlay – cast high noble metal, three or more surfaces
D6612	retainer onlay – cast predominantly base metal, two surfaces
D6613	retainer onlay – cast predominantly base metal, three or more surfaces
D6614	retainer onlay – cast noble metal, two surfaces
D6615	retainer onlay – cast noble metal, three or more surfaces
D6634	retainer onlay – titanium

Fixed Partial Denture Retainers – Crowns

D6710   **retainer crown – indirect resin based composite**
Not to be used as a temporary or provisional prosthesis.

D6720   **retainer crown – resin with high noble metal**

D6721   **retainer crown – resin with predominantly base metal**

D6722   **retainer crown – resin with noble metal**

D6740   **retainer crown – porcelain/ceramic**

D6750   **retainer crown – porcelain fused to high noble metal**

D6751   **retainer crown – porcelain fused to predominantly base metal**

D6752   **retainer crown – porcelain fused to noble metal**

D6753   **retainer crown – porcelain fused to titanium and titanium alloys**

D6780   **retainer crown – ¾ cast high noble metal**

D6781   **retainer crown – ¾ cast predominantly base metal**

D6782   **retainer crown – ¾ cast noble metal**

D6783   **retainer crown – ¾ porcelain/ceramic**

D6784   **retainer crown – ¾ titanium and titanium alloys**

D6790   **retainer crown – full cast high noble metal**

D6791   **retainer crown – full cast predominantly base metal**

D6792   **retainer crown – full cast noble metal**

D6794   **retainer crown – titanium and titanium alloys**

D6793   **interim retainer crown – further treatment or completion of diagnosis necessary prior to final impression**
Not to be used as a temporary retainer crown for a routine prosthetic restoration.

Other Fixed Partial Denture Services

D6920   **connector bar**
A device attached to fixed partial denture retainer or coping which serves to stabilize and anchor a removable overdenture prosthesis.

D6930   **re-cement or re-bond fixed partial denture**

D6940   **stress breaker**
A non-rigid connector.

D6950   **precision attachment**
A pair of components constitutes one precision attachment that is separate from the prosthesis.

D6980   **fixed partial denture repair necessitated by restorative material failure**

D6985   **pediatric partial denture, fixed**
This prosthesis is used primarily for aesthetic purposes.

D6999   **unspecified fixed prosthodontic procedure, by report**
Used for a procedure that is not adequately described by a code. Describe the procedure.

X. Oral & Maxillofacial Surgery

Local anesthesia is usually considered to be part of Oral and Maxillofacial Surgical procedures.

For dental benefit reporting purposes a quadrant is defined as four or more contiguous teeth and/or teeth spaces distal to the midline.

Extractions (Includes Local Anesthesia, Suturing If Needed, and Routine Postoperative Care)

D7111 **extraction, coronal remnants – primary tooth**
Removal of soft tissue-retained coronal remnants.

D7140 **extraction, erupted tooth or exposed root (elevation and/or forceps removal)**
Includes removal of tooth structure, minor smoothing of socket bone, and closure, as necessary.

D7210 **extraction, erupted tooth requiring removal of bone and/or sectioning of tooth, and including elevation of mucoperiosteal flap if indicated**
Includes related cutting of gingiva and bone, removal of tooth structure, minor smoothing of socket bone and closure.

D7220 **removal of impacted tooth – soft tissue**
Occlusal surface of tooth covered by soft tissue; requires mucoperiosteal flap elevation.

D7230 **removal of impacted tooth – partially bony**
Part of crown covered by bone; requires mucoperiosteal flap elevation and bone removal.

D7240 **removal of impacted tooth – completely bony**
Most or all of crown covered by bone; requires mucoperiosteal flap elevation and bone removal.

D7241 **removal of impacted tooth – completely bony, with unusual surgical complications**
Most or all of crown covered by bone; unusually difficult or complicated due to factors such as nerve dissection required, separate closure of maxillary sinus required or aberrant tooth position.

D7250 **removal of residual tooth roots (cutting procedure)**
Includes cutting of soft tissue and bone, removal of tooth structure, and closure.

D7251 **coronectomy – intentional partial tooth removal, impacted teeth only**
Intentional partial tooth removal is performed when a neurovascular complication is likely if the entire impacted tooth is removed.

Other Surgical Procedures

D7260 **oroantral fistula closure**
Excision of fistulous tract between maxillary sinus and oral cavity and closure by advancement flap.

D7261 **primary closure of a sinus perforation**
Subsequent to surgical removal of tooth, exposure of sinus requiring repair, or immediate closure of oroantral or oralnasal communication in absence of fistulous tract.

D7270 **tooth re-implantation and/or stabilization of accidentally evulsed or displaced tooth**
Includes splinting and/or stabilization.

D7272 **tooth transplantation (includes re-implantation from one site to another and splinting and/or stabilization)**

D7280 **exposure of an unerupted tooth**
An incision is made and the tissue is reflected and bone removed as necessary to expose the crown of an impacted tooth not intended to be extracted.

D7282 **mobilization of erupted or malpositioned tooth to aid eruption**
To move/luxate teeth to eliminate ankylosis; not in conjunction with an extraction.

D7283 **placement of device to facilitate eruption of impacted tooth**
Placement of an attachment on an unerupted tooth, after its exposure, to aid in its eruption. Report the surgical exposure separately using D7280.

● **D7284** **excisional biopsy of minor salivary glands**

D7285   **incisional biopsy of oral tissue – hard (bone, tooth)**
For partial removal of specimen only. This procedure involves biopsy of osseous lesions and is not used for apicoectomy/periradicular surgery. This procedure does not entail an excision.

D7286   **incisional biopsy of oral tissue – soft**
For partial removal of an architecturally intact specimen only. This procedure is not used at the same time as codes for apicoectomy/periradicular curettage. This procedure does not entail an excision.

D7287   **exfoliative cytological sample collection**
For collection of non-transepithelial cytology sample via mild scraping of the oral mucosa.

D7288   **brush biopsy – transepithelial sample collection**
For collection of oral disaggregated transepithelial cells via rotational brushing of the oral mucosa.

D7290   **surgical repositioning of teeth**
Grafting procedure(s) is/are additional.

D7291   **transseptal fiberotomy/supra crestal fiberotomy, by report**
The supraosseous connective tissue attachment is surgically severed around the involved teeth. Where there are adjacent teeth, the transseptal fiberotomy of a single tooth will involve a minimum of three teeth. Since the incisions are within the gingival sulcus and tissue and the root surface is not instrumented, this procedure heals by the reunion of connective tissue with the root surface on which viable periodontal tissue is present (reattachment).

D7292   **placement of temporary anchorage device [screw retained plate] requiring flap**

D7298   **removal of temporary anchorage device [screw retained plate], requiring flap**

D7293   **placement of temporary anchorage device requiring flap**

D7299   **removal of temporary anchorage device, requiring flap**

D7294   **placement of temporary anchorage device without flap**

D7300   **removal of temporary anchorage device without flap**

D7295   **harvest of bone for use in autogenous grafting procedure**
Reported in addition to those autogenous graft placement procedures that do not include harvesting of bone.

D7296   **corticotomy – one to three teeth or tooth spaces, per quadrant**
This procedure involves creating multiple cuts, perforations, or removal of cortical, alveolar or basal bone of the jaw for the purpose of facilitating orthodontic repositioning of the dentition. This procedure includes flap entry and closure. Graft material and membrane, if used, should be reported separately.

D7297   **corticotomy – four or more teeth or tooth spaces, per quadrant**
This procedure involves creating multiple cuts, perforations, or removal of cortical, alveolar or basal bone of the jaw for the purpose of facilitating orthodontic repositioning of the dentition. This procedure includes flap entry and closure. Graft material and membrane, if used, should be reported separately.

Alveoloplasty – Preparation of Ridge

D7310   **alveoloplasty in conjunction with extractions – four or more teeth or tooth spaces, per quadrant**
The alveoloplasty is distinct (separate procedure) from extractions. Usually in preparation for a prosthesis or other treatments such as radiation therapy and transplant surgery.

D7311   **alveoloplasty in conjunction with extractions – one to three teeth or tooth spaces, per quadrant**
The alveoloplasty is distinct (separate procedure) from extractions. Usually in preparation for a prosthesis or other treatments such as radiation therapy and transplant surgery.

D7320   **alveoloplasty not in conjunction with extractions – four or more teeth or tooth spaces, per quadrant**
No extractions performed in an edentulous area. See D7310 if teeth are being extracted concurrently with the alveoloplasty. Usually in preparation for a prosthesis or other treatments such as radiation therapy and transplant surgery.

D7321   **alveoloplasty not in conjunction with extractions – one to three teeth or tooth spaces, per quadrant**
No extractions performed in an edentulous area. See D7311 if teeth are being extracted concurrently with the alveoloplasty. Usually in preparation for a prosthesis or other treatments such as radiation therapy and transplant surgery.

Vestibuloplasty

Any of a series of surgical procedures designed to increase relative alveolar ridge height.

D7340 **vestibuloplasty – ridge extension (secondary epithelialization)**

D7350 **vestibuloplasty – ridge extension (including soft tissue grafts, muscle reattachment, revision of soft tissue attachment and management of hypertrophied and hyperplastic tissue)**

Excision of Soft Tissue Lesions

Includes non-odontogenic cysts.

D7410 **excision of benign lesion up to 1.25 cm**

D7411 **excision of benign lesion greater than 1.25 cm**

D7412 **excision of benign lesion, complicated**
Requires extensive undermining with advancement or rotational flap closure.

D7413 **excision of malignant lesion up to 1.25 cm**

D7414 **excision of malignant lesion greater than 1.25 cm**

D7415 **excision of malignant lesion, complicated**
Requires extensive undermining with advancement or rotational flap closure.

D7465 **destruction of lesion(s) by physical or chemical method, by report**
Examples include using cryo, laser or electro surgery.

Excision of Intra-Osseous Lesions

D7440 **excision of malignant tumor – lesion diameter up to 1.25 cm**

D7441 **excision of malignant tumor – lesion diameter greater than 1.25 cm**

D7450 **removal of benign odontogenic cyst or tumor – lesion diameter up to 1.25 cm**

D7451 **removal of benign odontogenic cyst or tumor – lesion diameter greater than 1.25 cm**

D7460 **removal of benign nonodontogenic cyst or tumor – lesion diameter up to 1.25 cm**

D7461 **removal of benign nonodontogenic cyst or tumor – lesion diameter greater than 1.25 cm**

Excision of Bone Tissue

D7471   **removal of lateral exostosis (maxilla or mandible)**

D7472   **removal of torus palatinus**

D7473   **removal of torus mandibularis**

D7485   **reduction of osseous tuberosity**

D7490   **radical resection of maxilla or mandible**
Partial resection of maxilla or mandible; removal of lesion and defect with margin of normal appearing bone. Reconstruction and bone grafts should be reported separately.

Surgical Incision

D7509   **marsupialization of odontogenic cyst**
Surgical decompression of a large cystic lesion by creating a long-term open pocket or pouch.

D7510   **incision and drainage of abscess – intraoral soft tissue**
Involves incision through mucosa, including periodontal origins.

D7511   **incision and drainage of abscess – intraoral soft tissue – complicated (includes drainage of multiple fascial spaces)**
Incision is made intraorally and dissection is extended into adjacent fascial space(s) to provide adequate drainage of abscess/cellulitis.

D7520   **incision and drainage of abscess – extraoral soft tissue**
Involves incision through skin.

D7521   **incision and drainage of abscess – extraoral soft tissue – complicated (includes drainage of multiple fascial spaces)**
Incision is made extraorally and dissection is extended into adjacent fascial space(s) to provide adequate drainage of abscess/cellulitis.

D7530   **removal of foreign body from mucosa, skin, or subcutaneous alveolar tissue**

D7540   **removal of reaction producing foreign bodies, musculoskeletal system**
May include, but is not limited to, removal of splinters, pieces of wire, etc., from muscle and/or bone.

D7550   **partial ostectomy/sequestrectomy for removal of non-vital bone**
Removal of loose or sloughed-off dead bone caused by infection or reduced blood supply.

D7560   **maxillary sinusotomy for removal of tooth fragment or foreign body**

Treatment of Closed Fractures

D7610   **maxilla – open reduction (teeth immobilized, if present)**
Teeth may be wired, banded or splinted together to prevent movement. Incision required for interosseous fixation.

D7620   **maxilla – closed reduction (teeth immobilized, if present)**
No incision required to reduce fracture. See D7610 if interosseous fixation is applied.

D7630   **mandible – open reduction (teeth immobilized, if present)**
Teeth may be wired, banded or splinted together to prevent movement. Incision required to reduce fracture.

D7640   **mandible – closed reduction (teeth immobilized, if present)**
No incision required to reduce fracture. See D7630 if interosseous fixation is applied.

D7650   **malar and/or zygomatic arch – open reduction**

D7660   **malar and/or zygomatic arch – closed reduction**

D7670   **alveolus – closed reduction, may include stabilization of teeth**
Teeth may be wired, banded or splinted together to prevent movement.

D7671   **alveolus – open reduction, may include stabilization of teeth**
Teeth may be wired, banded or splinted together to prevent movement.

D7680   **facial bones – complicated reduction with fixation and multiple surgical approaches**
Facial bones include upper and lower jaw, cheek, and bones around eyes, nose, and ears.

Treatment of Open Fractures

D7710   **maxilla – open reduction**
Incision required to reduce fracture.

D7720   **maxilla – closed reduction**

D7730   **mandible – open reduction**
Incision required to reduce fracture.

Section 1: Code on Dental Procedures and Nomenclature

D7740   **mandible – closed reduction**

D7750   **malar and/or zygomatic arch – open reduction**
Incision required to reduce fracture.

D7760   **malar and/or zygomatic arch – closed reduction**

D7770   **alveolus – open reduction stabilization of teeth**
Fractured bone(s) are exposed to mouth or outside the face.
Incision required to reduce fracture.

D7771   **alveolus, closed reduction stabilization of teeth**
Fractured bone(s) are exposed to mouth or outside the face.

D7780   **facial bones – complicated reduction with fixation and multiple approaches**
Incision required to reduce fracture. Facial bones include upper and lower jaw, cheek, and bones around eyes, nose, and ears.

Reduction of Dislocation and Management of Other Temporomandibular Joint Dysfunctions

Procedures that are an integral part of a primary procedure should not be reported separately.

D7810   **open reduction of dislocation**
Access to TMJ via surgical opening.

D7820   **closed reduction of dislocation**
Joint manipulated into place; no surgical exposure.

D7830   **manipulation under anesthesia**
Usually done under general anesthesia or intravenous sedation.

D7840   **condylectomy**
Removal of all or portion of the mandibular condyle (separate procedure).

D7850   **surgical discectomy, with/without implant**
Excision of the intra-articular disc of a joint.

D7852   **disc repair**
Repositioning and/or sculpting of disc; repair of perforated posterior attachment.

D7854   **synovectomy**
Excision of a portion or all of the synovial membrane of a joint.

● new procedure code   ▲ revision to a nomenclature or descriptor   # editorial

D7856 **myotomy**
Cutting of muscle for therapeutic purposes (separate procedure).

D7858 **joint reconstruction**
Reconstruction of osseous components including or excluding soft tissues of the joint with autogenous, homologous, or alloplastic materials.

D7860 **arthrotomy**
Cutting into joint (separate procedure).

D7865 **arthroplasty**
Reduction of osseous components of the joint to create a pseudoarthrosis or eliminate an irregular remodeling pattern (osteophytes).

D7870 **arthrocentesis**
Withdrawal of fluid from a joint space by aspiration.

D7871 **non-arthroscopic lysis and lavage**
Inflow and outflow catheters are placed into the joint space. The joint is lavaged and manipulated as indicated in an effort to release minor adhesions and synovial vacuum phenomenon as well as to remove inflammation products from the joint space.

D7872 **arthroscopy – diagnosis, with or without biopsy**

D7873 **arthroscopy: lavage and lysis of adhesions**
Removal of adhesions using the arthroscope and lavage of the joint cavities.

D7874 **arthroscopy: disc repositioning and stabilization**
Repositioning and stabilization of disc using arthroscopic techniques.

D7875 **arthroscopy: synovectomy**
Removal of inflamed and hyperplastic synovium (partial/complete) via an arthroscopic technique.

D7876 **arthroscopy: discectomy**
Removal of disc and remodeled posterior attachment via the arthroscope.

D7877 **arthroscopy: debridement**
Removal of pathologic hard and/or soft tissue using the arthroscope.

D7880 **occlusal orthotic device, by report**
Presently includes splints provided for treatment of temporomandibular joint dysfunction.

D7881 **occlusal orthotic device adjustment**

D7899   **unspecified TMD therapy, by report**
Used for procedure that is not adequately described by a code.
Describe procedure.

Repair of Traumatic Wounds

Excludes closure of surgical incisions.

D7910   **suture of recent small wounds up to 5 cm**

Complicated Suturing (Reconstruction Requiring Delicate Handling of Tissues and Wide Undermining for Meticulous Closure)

Excludes closure of surgical incisions.

D7911   **complicated suture – up to 5 cm**

D7912   **complicated suture – greater than 5 cm**

Other Repair Procedures

D7920   **skin graft (identify defect covered, location and type of graft)**

D7921   **collection and application of autologous blood concentrate product**

D7922   **placement of intra-socket biological dressing to aid in hemostasis or clot stabilization, per site**
This procedure can be performed at time and/or after extraction to aid in hemostasis. The socket is packed with a hemostatic agent to aid in hemostasis and or clot stabilization.

D7940   **osteoplasty – for orthognathic deformities**
Reconstruction of jaws for correction of congenital, developmental or acquired traumatic or surgical deformity.

● **D7939**   **indexing for osteotomy using dynamic robotic assisted or dynamic navigation**
A guide is stabilized to the teeth and/or the bone to allow for virtual guidance of osteotomy.

D7941   **osteotomy – mandibular rami**

D7943   **osteotomy – mandibular rami with bone graft; includes obtaining the graft**

D7944 **osteotomy – segmented or subapical**
Report by range of tooth numbers within segment.

D7945 **osteotomy – body of mandible**
Sectioning of lower jaw. This includes the exposure, bone cut, fixation, routine wound closure and normal post-operative follow-up care.

D7946 **LeFort I (maxilla – total)**
Sectioning of the upper jaw. This includes exposure, bone cuts, downfracture, repositioning, fixation, routine wound closure and normal post-operative follow-up care.

D7947 **LeFort I (maxilla – segmented)**
When reporting a surgically assisted palatal expansion without downfracture, this code would entail a reduced service and should be "by report."

D7948 **LeFort II or LeFort III (osteoplasty of facial bones for midface hypoplasia or retrusion) – without bone graft**
Sectioning of upper jaw. This includes exposure, bone cuts, downfracture, segmentation of maxilla, repositioning, fixation, routine wound closure and normal post-operative follow-up care.

D7949 **LeFort II or LeFort III – with bone graft**
Includes obtaining autografts.

D7950 **osseous, osteoperiosteal, or cartilage graft of the mandible or maxilla – autogenous or nonautogenous, by report**
This procedure is for ridge augmentation or reconstruction to increase height, width and/or volume of residual alveolar ridge. It includes obtaining graft material. Placement of a barrier membrane, if used, should be reported separately.

D7951 **sinus augmentation with bone or bone substitutes via a lateral open approach**
The augmentation of the sinus cavity to increase alveolar height for reconstruction of edentulous portions of the maxilla. This procedure is performed via a lateral open approach. This includes obtaining the bone or bone substitutes. Placement of a barrier membrane if used should be reported separately.

D7952 **sinus augmentation via a vertical approach**
The augmentation of the sinus to increase alveolar height by vertical access through the ridge crest by raising the floor of the sinus and grafting as necessary. This includes obtaining the bone or bone substitutes.

D7953   **bone replacement graft for ridge preservation – per site**
Graft is placed in an extraction or implant removal site at the time of the extraction or removal to preserve ridge integrity (e.g., clinically indicated in preparation for implant reconstruction or where alveolar contour is critical to planned prosthetic reconstruction). Does not include obtaining graft material. Membrane, if used should be reported separately.

D7955   **repair of maxillofacial soft and/or hard tissue defect**
Reconstruction of surgical, traumatic, or congenital defects of the facial bones, including the mandible, may utilize graft materials in conjunction with soft tissue procedures to repair and restore the facial bones to form and function. This does not include obtaining the graft and these procedures may require multiple surgical approaches. This procedure does not include edentulous maxilla and mandibular reconstruction for prosthetic considerations.

D7956   **guided tissue regeneration, edentulous area – resorbable barrier, per site**
This procedure does not include flap entry and closure, or, when indicated, wound debridement, osseous contouring, bone replacement grafts, and placement of biologic materials to aid in osseous regeneration. This procedure may be used for ridge augmentation, sinus lift procedures, and after tooth extraction.

D7957   **guided tissue regeneration, edentulous area – non-resorbable barrier, per site**
This procedure does not include flap entry and closure, or, when indicated, wound debridement, osseous contouring, bone replacement grafts, and placement of biologic materials to aid in osseous regeneration. This procedure may be used for ridge augmentation, sinus lift procedures, and after tooth extraction.

D7961   **buccal / labial frenectomy (frenulectomy)**

D7962   **lingual frenectomy (frenulectomy)**

D7963   **frenuloplasty**
Excision of frenum with accompanying excision or repositioning of aberrant muscle and z-plasty or other local flap closure.

D7970   **excision of hyperplastic tissue – per arch**

D7971   **excision of pericoronal gingiva**
Removal of inflammatory or hypertrophied tissues surrounding partially erupted/impacted teeth.

D7972   **surgical reduction of fibrous tuberosity**

D7979   **non – surgical sialolithotomy**
A sialolith is removed from the gland or ductal portion of the gland without surgical incision into the gland or the duct of the gland; for example via manual manipulation, ductal dilation, or any other non-surgical method.

D7980   **surgical sialolithotomy**
Procedure by which a stone within a salivary gland or its duct is removed, either intraorally or extraorally.

D7981   **excision of salivary gland, by report**

D7982   **sialodochoplasty**
Procedure for the repair of a defect and/or restoration of a portion of a salivary gland duct.

D7983   **closure of salivary fistula**
Closure of an opening between a salivary duct and/or gland and the cutaneous surface, or an opening into the oral cavity through other than the normal anatomic pathway.

D7990   **emergency tracheotomy**
Formation of a tracheal opening usually below the cricoid cartilage to allow for respiratory exchange.

D7991   **coronoidectomy**
Removal of the coronoid process of the mandible.

D7993   **surgical placement of craniofacial implant – extra oral**
Surgical placement of a craniofacial implant to aid in retention of an auricular, nasal, or orbital prosthesis.

D7994   **surgical placement: zygomatic implant**
An implant placed in the zygomatic bone and exiting through the maxillary mucosal tissue providing support and attachment of a maxillary dental prosthesis.

D7995   **synthetic graft – mandible or facial bones, by report**
Includes allogenic material.

D7996   implant-mandible for augmentation purposes (excluding alveolar ridge), by report

D7997   appliance removal (not by dentist who placed appliance), includes removal of archbar

D7998   intraoral placement of a fixation device not in conjunction with a fracture

The placement of intermaxillary fixation appliance for documented medically accepted treatments not in association with fractures.

D7999   unspecified oral surgery procedure, by report

Used for a procedure that is not adequately described by a code. Describe the procedure.

XI. Orthodontics

All of the following orthodontic treatment codes may be used more than once for the treatment of a particular patient depending on the particular circumstance. A patient may require more than one limited or comprehensive procedure depending on their particular problems.

Dentition

Primary Dentition: Teeth developed and erupted first in order of time.

Transitional Dentition: The final phase of the transition from primary to adult teeth, in which the deciduous molars and canines are in the process of shedding and the permanent successors are emerging.

Adolescent Dentition: The dentition that is present after the normal loss of primary teeth and prior to cessation of growth that would affect orthodontic treatment.

Adult Dentition: The dentition that is present after the cessation of growth that would affect orthodontic treatment.

Limited Orthodontic Treatment

Orthodontic treatment utilizing any therapeutic modality with a limited objective or scale of treatment. Treatment may occur in any stage of dental development or dentition.

The objective may be limited by:

- not involving the entire dentition.

- not attempting to address the full scope of the existing or developing orthodontic problem.

- mitigating an aspect of a greater malocclusion (i.e. crossbite, overjet, overbite, arch length, anterior alignment, one phase of multi-phase treatment, treatment prior to the permanent dentition, etc.).

- a decision to defer or forego comprehensive treatment.

D8010   **limited orthodontic treatment of the primary dentition**

D8020   **limited orthodontic treatment of the transitional dentition**

D8030   **limited orthodontic treatment of the adolescent dentition**

D8040   **limited orthodontic treatment of the adult dentition**

Comprehensive Orthodontic Treatment

Comprehensive orthodontic care includes a coordinated diagnosis and treatment leading to the improvement of a patient's craniofacial dysfunction and/or dentofacial deformity which may include anatomical, functional and/or aesthetic relationships. Treatment may utilize fixed and/or removable orthodontic appliances and may also include functional and/or orthopedic appliances in growing and non-growing patients. Adjunctive procedures to facilitate care may be required. Comprehensive orthodontics may incorporate treatment phases focusing on specific objectives at various stages of dentofacial development.

D8070 **comprehensive orthodontic treatment of the transitional dentition**

D8080 **comprehensive orthodontic treatment of the adolescent dentition**

D8090 **comprehensive orthodontic treatment of the adult dentition**

Minor Treatment to Control Harmful Habits

D8210 **removable appliance therapy**
Removable indicates patient can remove; includes appliances for thumb sucking and tongue thrusting.

D8220 **fixed appliance therapy**
Fixed indicates patient cannot remove appliance; includes appliances for thumb sucking and tongue thrusting.

Other Orthodontic Services

D8660 **pre-orthodontic treatment examination to monitor growth and development**
Periodic observation of patient dentition, at intervals established by the dentist, to determine when orthodontic treatment should begin. Diagnostic procedures are documented separately.

D8670 **periodic orthodontic treatment visit**

D8680 **orthodontic retention (removal of appliances, construction and placement of retainer(s))**

D8681 **removable orthodontic retainer adjustment**

D8695 **removal of fixed orthodontic appliances for reasons other than completion of treatment**

D8696   **repair of orthodontic appliance – maxillary**
Does not include bracket and standard fixed orthodontic appliances.
It does include functional appliances and palatal expanders.

D8697   **repair of orthodontic appliance – mandibular**
Does not include bracket and standard fixed orthodontic appliances.
It does include functional appliances and palatal expanders.

D8698   **re-cement or re-bond fixed retainer – maxillary**

D8699   **re-cement or re-bond fixed retainer – mandibular**

D8701   **repair of fixed retainer, includes reattachment – maxillary**

D8702   **repair of fixed retainer, includes reattachment – mandibular**

D8703   **replacement of lost or broken retainer – maxillary**

D8704   **replacement of lost or broken retainer – mandibular**

D8999   **unspecified orthodontic procedure, by report**
Used for a procedure that is not adequately described by a code.
Describe the procedure.

XII. Adjunctive General Services

Unclassified Treatment

D9110 **palliative treatment of dental pain – per visit**
Treatment that relieves pain but is not curative; services provided do not have distinct procedure codes.

D9120 **fixed partial denture sectioning**
Separation of one or more connections between abutments and/or pontics when some portion of a fixed prosthesis is to remain intact and serviceable following sectioning and extraction or other treatment. Includes all recontouring and polishing of retained portions.

D9130 **temporomandibular joint dysfunction – non-invasive physical therapies**
Therapy including but not limited to massage, diathermy, ultrasound, or cold application to provide relief from muscle spasms, inflammation or pain, intending to improve freedom of motion and joint function. This should be reported on a per session basis.

Anesthesia

D9210 **local anesthesia not in conjunction with operative or surgical procedures**

D9211 **regional block anesthesia**

D9212 **trigeminal division block anesthesia**

D9215 **local anesthesia in conjunction with operative or surgical procedures**

D9219 **evaluation for moderate sedation, deep sedation or general anesthesia**

D9222 **deep sedation/general anesthesia – first 15 minutes**
Anesthesia time begins when the doctor administering the anesthetic agent initiates the appropriate anesthesia and non-invasive monitoring protocol and remains in continuous attendance of the patient. Anesthesia services are considered completed when the patient may be safely left under the observation of trained personnel and the doctor may safely leave the room to attend to other patients or duties.

The level of anesthesia is determined by the anesthesia provider's documentation of the anesthetic effects upon the central nervous system and not dependent upon the route of administration.

D9223 **deep sedation/general anesthesia – each subsequent 15 minute increment**

D9230 **inhalation of nitrous oxide/analgesia, anxiolysis**

D9239 **intravenous moderate (conscious) sedation/analgesia – first 15 minutes**
Anesthesia time begins when the doctor administering the anesthetic agent initiates the appropriate anesthesia and non-invasive monitoring protocol and remains in continuous attendance of the patient. Anesthesia services are considered completed when the patient may be safely left under the observation of trained personnel and the doctor may safely leave the room to attend to other patients or duties.

The level of anesthesia is determined by the anesthesia provider's documentation of the anesthetic effects upon the central nervous system and not dependent upon the route of administration.

D9243 **intravenous moderate (conscious) sedation/analgesia – each subsequent 15 minute increment**

D9248 **non-intravenous conscious sedation**
This includes non-IV minimal and moderate sedation.

A medically controlled state of depressed consciousness while maintaining the patient's airway, protective reflexes and the ability to respond to stimulation or verbal commands. It includes non-intravenous administration of sedative and/or analgesic agent(s) and appropriate monitoring.

The level of anesthesia is determined by the anesthesia provider's documentation of the anesthetic's effects upon the central nervous system and not dependent upon the route of administration.

Professional Consultation

D9310 **consultation – diagnostic service provided by dentist or physician other than requesting dentist or physician**
A patient encounter with a practitioner whose opinion or advice regarding evaluation and/or management of a specific problem; may be requested by another practitioner or appropriate source. The consultation includes an oral evaluation. The consulted practitioner may initiate diagnostic and/or therapeutic services.

D9311 **consultation with a medical health care professional**
Treating dentist consults with a medical health care professional concerning medical issues that may affect patient's planned dental treatment.

Professional Visits

D9410   **house/extended care facility call**
Includes visits to nursing homes, long-term care facilities, hospice sites, institutions, etc. Report in addition to reporting appropriate code numbers for actual services performed.

D9420   **hospital or ambulatory surgical center call**
Care provided outside the dentist's office to a patient who is in a hospital or ambulatory surgical center. Services delivered to the patient on the date of service are documented separately using the applicable procedure codes.

D9430   **office visit for observation (during regularly scheduled hours) – no other services performed**

D9440   **office visit – after regularly scheduled hours**

D9450   **case presentation, subsequent to detailed and extensive treatment planning**

Drugs

D9610   **therapeutic parenteral drug, single administration**
Includes single administration of antibiotics, steroids, anti-inflammatory drugs, or other therapeutic medications. This code should not be used to report administration of sedative, anesthetic or reversal agents.

D9612   **therapeutic parenteral drugs, two or more administrations, different medications**
Includes multiple administrations of antibiotics, steroids, anti-inflammatory drugs or other therapeutic medications. This code should not be used to report administration of sedatives, anesthetic or reversal agents.

This code should be reported when two or more different medications are necessary and should not be reported in addition to code D9610 on the same date.

D9613   **infiltration of sustained release therapeutic drug, per quadrant**
Infiltration of a sustained release pharmacologic agent for long acting surgical site pain control. Not for local anesthesia purposes.

D9630   **drugs or medicaments dispensed in the office for home use**
Includes, but is not limited to oral antibiotics, oral analgesics, and topical fluoride; does not include writing prescriptions.

Miscellaneous Services

D9910 **application of desensitizing medicament**
Includes in-office treatment for root sensitivity. Typically reported on a "per visit" basis for application of topical fluoride. This code is not to be used for bases, liners or adhesives used under restorations.

D9911 **application of desensitizing resin for cervical and/or root surface, per tooth**
Typically reported on a "per tooth" basis for application of adhesive resins. This code is not to be used for bases, liners, or adhesives used under restorations.

D9912 **pre-visit patient screening**
Capture and documentation of a patient's health status prior to or on the scheduled date of service to evaluate risk of infectious disease transmission if the patient is to be treated within the dental practice.

D9920 **behavior management, by report**
May be reported in addition to treatment provided. Should be reported in 15-minute increments.

D9930 **treatment of complications (post-surgical) – unusual circumstances, by report**
For example, treatment of a dry socket following extraction or removal of bony sequestrum.

D9932 **cleaning and inspection of removable complete denture, maxillary**
This procedure does not include any adjustments.

D9933 **cleaning and inspection of removable complete denture, mandibular**
This procedure does not include any adjustments.

D9934 **cleaning and inspection of removable partial denture, maxillary**
This procedure does not include any adjustments.

D9935 **cleaning and inspection of removable partial denture, mandibular**
This procedure does not include any adjustments.

● **D9938** **fabrication of a custom removable clear plastic temporary aesthetic appliance**

● **D9939** **placement of a custom removable clear plastic temporary aesthetic appliance**

D9941 **fabrication of athletic mouthguard**

Section 1: Code on Dental Procedures and Nomenclature

D9942   **repair and/or reline of occlusal guard**

D9943   **occlusal guard adjustment**

D9944   **occlusal guard – hard appliance, full arch**
Removable dental appliance designed to minimize the effects of bruxism or other occlusal factors. Not to be reported for any type of sleep apnea, snoring or TMD appliances.

D9945   **occlusal guard – soft appliance, full arch**
Removable dental appliance designed to minimize the effects of bruxism or other occlusal factors. Not to be reported for any type of sleep apnea, snoring or TMD appliances.

D9946   **occlusal guard – hard appliance, partial arch**
Removable dental appliance designed to minimize the effects of bruxism or other occlusal factors. Provides only partial occlusal coverage such as anterior deprogrammer. Not to be reported for any type of sleep apnea, snoring or TMD appliances.

D9950   **occlusion analysis – mounted case**
Includes, but is not limited to, facebow, interocclusal records tracings, and diagnostic wax-up; for diagnostic casts, see D0470.

D9951   **occlusal adjustment – limited**
May also be known as equilibration; reshaping the occlusal surfaces of teeth to create harmonious contact relationships between the maxillary and mandibular teeth. Presently includes discing/odontoplasty/enamoplasty. Typically reported on a "per visit" basis. This should not be reported when the procedure only involves bite adjustment in the routine post-delivery care for a direct/indirect restoration or fixed/removable prosthodontics.

D9952   **occlusal adjustment – complete**
Occlusal adjustment may require several appointments of varying length, and sedation may be necessary to attain adequate relaxation of the musculature. Study casts mounted on an articulating instrument may be utilized for analysis of occlusal disharmony. It is designed to achieve functional relationships and masticatory efficiency in conjunction with restorative treatment, orthodontics, orthognathic surgery, or jaw trauma when indicated. Occlusal adjustment enhances the healing potential of tissues affected by the lesions of occlusal trauma.

D9970 **enamel microabrasion**
The removal of discolored surface enamel defects resulting from altered mineralization or decalcification of the superficial enamel layer. Submit per treatment visit.

D9971 **odontoplasty – per tooth**
Removal/reshaping of enamel surfaces or projections.

D9972 **external bleaching – per arch – performed in office**

D9973 **external bleaching – per tooth**

D9974 **internal bleaching – per tooth**

D9975 **external bleaching for home application, per arch; includes materials and fabrication of custom trays**

Non-clinical procedures

D9961 **duplicate/copy patient's records**

D9985 **sales tax**

D9986 **missed appointment**

D9987 **cancelled appointment**

D9990 **certified translation or sign-language services – per visit**

D9991 **dental case management – addressing appointment compliance barriers**
Individualized efforts to assist a patient to maintain scheduled appointments by solving transportation challenges or other barriers.

D9992 **dental case management – care coordination**
Assisting in a patient's decisions regarding the coordination of oral health care services across multiple providers, provider types, specialty areas of treatment, health care settings, health care organizations and payment systems. This is the additional time and resources expended to provide experience or expertise beyond that possessed by the patient.

D9993 **dental case management – motivational interviewing**
Patient-centered, personalized counseling using methods such as Motivational Interviewing (MI) to identify and modify behaviors interfering with positive oral health outcomes. This is a separate service from traditional nutritional or tobacco counseling.

D9994 **dental case management – patient education to improve oral health literacy**
Individual, customized communication of information to assist the patient in making appropriate health decisions designed to improve oral health literacy, explained in a manner acknowledging economic circumstances and different cultural beliefs, values, attitudes, traditions and language preferences, and adopting information and services to these differences, which requires the expenditure of time and resources beyond that of an oral evaluation or case presentation.

D9997 **dental case management – patients with special health care needs**
Special treatment considerations for patients/individuals with physical, medical, developmental or cognitive conditions resulting in substantial functional limitations or incapacitation, which require that modifications be made to delivery of treatment to provide customized or comprehensive oral health care services.

D9995 **teledentistry – synchronous; real-time encounter**
Reported in addition to other procedures (e.g., diagnostic) delivered to the patient on the date of service.

D9996 **teledentistry – asynchronous; information stored and forwarded to dentist for subsequent review**
Reported in addition to other procedures (e.g., diagnostic) delivered to the patient on the date of service.

D9999 **unspecified adjunctive procedure, by report**
Used for a procedure that is not adequately described by a code. Describe the procedure.

• XIII. Sleep Apnea Services

D9947   **custom sleep apnea appliance fabrication and placement**

D9948   **adjustment of custom sleep apnea appliance**

D9949   **repair of custom sleep apnea appliance**

D9953   **reline custom sleep apnea appliance (indirect)**
Resurface dentition side of appliance with new soft or hard base material as required to restore original form and function.

• **D9954**   **fabrication and delivery of oral appliance therapy (OAT) morning repositioning device**
Device for use immediately after removing a mandibular advancement device to aid in relieving muscle/jaw pain and occlusal changes.

• **D9955**   **oral appliance therapy (OAT) titration visit**
Post-delivery visit for titration of a mandibular advancement device and to subsequently evaluate the patient's response to treatment, integrity of the device, and management of side effects.

• **D9956**   **administration of home sleep apnea test**
Sleep apnea test, for patients who are at risk for sleep related breathing disorders and appropriate candidates, as allowed by applicable laws. Also to help the dentist in defining the optimal position of the mandible.

• **D9957**   **screening for sleep related breathing disorders**
Screening activities, performed alone or in conjunction with another evaluation, to identify signs and symptoms of sleep-related breathing disorders.

Section 2
CDT Code Changes Markup

This CDT Code version is effective January 1, 2024 through December 31, 2024. All changes are illustrated in this section, color-coded as follows:

- Additions will be in blue ink without underlining

- Deletions will be stricken through in red ink

- Revisions and Editorial changes will have added text underlined in blue ink and deleted text stricken through in red ink.

There are:

- 15 Additions (count includes fourteen [14] new codes and one [1] new category of service, Sleep Apnea Services)

- 2 Revisions

- 0 Deletions

- 0 Editorial (e.g., syntax; spelling) actions that clarify without changing the CDT Code entry's purpose or scope

As noted in the Preface, the CDT Code is presented in several groupings identified as Categories of Service and, within each, one or more subcategories (etc.) to organize the content. This presentation structure, in addition to the manual's alphabetic and numeric indices, are aids to finding the applicable code to document and report a procedure delivered to a patient.

Classification of Materials

Additions
None

Revisions
None

Deletions
None

Editorial
None

I. Diagnostic

Additions
One (1) entry

Post Processing of Image or Image Sets

   D0396 **3D printing of a 3D dental surface scan**
          3D printing of a 3D dental surface scan to obtain a physical model.

Revisions
None

Deletions
None

Editorial
None

II. Preventive

Additions
One (1) entry

Other Preventive Services

D1301   immunization counseling
A review of a patient's vaccine and medical history, discussion of the vaccine benefits, risks, and consequences of not obtaining the vaccination. Counseling also includes a discussion of questions and concerns the patient, family, or caregiver may have and suggestions on where the patient can obtain the vaccine.

Revisions
None

Deletions
None

Editorial
None

III. Restorative

Additions
Three (3) entries

Other Restorative Services

D2976   **band stabilization – per tooth**
A band, typically cemented around a molar tooth after a multi-surface restoration is placed, to add support and resistance to fracture until a patient is ready for the full cuspal coverage restoration.

D2989   **excavation of a tooth resulting in the determination of non-restorability**

D2991   **application of hydroxyapatite regeneration medicament – per tooth**
Preparation of tooth surfaces and topical application of a scaffold to guide hydroxyapatite regeneration.

Revisions
One (1) entry

Resin-Based Composite Restorations – Direct

D2335   **resin-based composite – four or more surfaces** ~~or involving incisal angle~~ **(anterior)**
~~Incisal angle to be defined as one of the angles formed by the junction of the incisal and the mesial or distal surface of an anterior tooth.~~

Deletions
None

Editorial
None

Section 2: CDT Code Changes Markup

IV. Endodontics

Additions
None

Revisions
None

Deletions
None

Editorial
None

V. Periodontics

Additions
None

Revisions
None

Deletions
None

Editorial
None

VI. Prosthodontics, removable

Additions
None

Revisions
One (1) entry

Other Removable Prosthetic Services

D5876 add metal substructure to acrylic full denture (per arch)
Use of metal substructure in removable complete dentures without a framework.

Deletions
None

Editorial
None

VII. Maxillofacial Prosthetics

Additions
None

Revisions
None

Deletions
None

Editorial
None

VIII. Implant Services

Additions
One (1) entry

Other Implant Services

D6089   accessing and retorquing loose implant screw – per screw

Revisions
None

Deletions
None

Editorial
None

IX. Prosthodontics, fixed

Additions
None

Revisions
None

Deletions
None

Editorial
None

X. Oral & Maxillofacial Surgery

Additions
Two (2) entries

Other Surgical Procedures

D7284   excisional biopsy of minor salivary glands

Other Repair Procedures

D7939   indexing for osteotomy using dynamic robotic assisted or dynamic navigation
A guide is stabilized to the teeth and/or the bone to allow for virtual guidance of osteotomy.

Revisions
None

Deletions
None

Editorial
None

XI. Orthodontics

Additions
None

Revisions
None

Deletions
None

Editorial
None

XII. Adjunctive General Services

Additions

Two (2) entries

Miscellaneous Services

D9938 fabrication of a custom removable clear plastic temporary aesthetic appliance

D9939 placement of a custom removable clear plastic temporary aesthetic appliance

Revisions

None

Deletions

None

Editorial

None

XIII. Sleep Apnea Services

Note: This category was added in CDT 2024 and also includes current codes D9947, D9948, D9949, and D9953.

Additions
Four (4) entries

D9954 **fabrication and delivery of oral appliance therapy (OAT) morning repositioning device**
Device for use immediately after removing a mandibular advancement device to aid in relieving muscle/jaw pain and occlusal changes.

D9955 **oral appliance therapy (OAT) titration visit**
Post-delivery visit for titration of a mandibular advancement device and to subsequently evaluate the patient's response to treatment, integrity of the device, and management of side effects.

D9956 **administration of home sleep apnea test**
Sleep apnea test, for patients who are at risk for sleep related breathing disorders and appropriate candidates, as allowed by applicable laws. Also to help the dentist in defining the optimal position of the mandible.

D9957 **screening for sleep related breathing disorders**
Screening activities, performed alone or in conjunction with another evaluation, to identify signs and symptoms of sleep-related breathing disorders.

Revisions
None

Deletions
None

Editorial
None

Section 3

ICD-10-CM Diagnoses for Dental Diseases and Conditions

Table of Contents

ICD-10-CM Preface

Dentists, by virtue of their clinical education, experience, and professional ethics, are the individuals responsible for diagnosis. As such, a dentist is also obligated to select the appropriate diagnosis code for patient records and claim submission.

Both the ADA Dental Claim Form and the HIPAA standard electronic dental claim transaction are able to report up to four diagnosis codes. This capability was added to the claim forms with the expectation that ICD (International Classification of Diseases) would, at some point, become a required data element for dental claim adjudication.

Note: Guidance on reporting ICD codes on dental claims is found in the ADA Dental Claim Form's comprehensive completion instructions. The ICD coding instructions apply to three data items:

29a – **Diagnosis Code Pointer** ("A" through "D" as applicable from Item 34a)

34 – **Diagnosis Code List Qualifier** ("AB" for ICD-10-CM)

34a – **Diagnosis Code(s) / A, B, C, D** (Up to four, with the primary diagnosis adjacent to the letter "A")

These instructions are available online at *ADA.org/en/publications/cdt/ada-dental-claim-form*.

Federal regulations published under the auspices of HIPAA's Administrative Simplification provisions specify only ICD codes as valid on claim submissions.

Note: There is no immediate and universal mandate to include an ICD-10-CM code on all dental claims. Dental benefit plans are unlikely to establish identical diagnostic code reporting requirements. You should check with each plan for its requirements.

ICD-10-CM became the HIPAA standard on October 1, 2015. It is a code set maintained by the Federal government via an interdepartmental committee comprised of representatives from the Centers for Medicare and Medicaid Services (CMS) and the Centers for Disease Control and Prevention (CDC). Versions are published annually and are effective on October 1st. The complete and current code set is available online at: *www.cms.gov/Medicare/Coding/ICD10*.

Note: ICD-10-CM does not have a chapter for dentistry-only codes. The CDT manual contains a subset of the complete code set and contains entries identified by ADA member dentists appointed to the Council on Dental Benefit Programs as pertinent to most encounters and services provided to a dentist's patient.

Many diagnoses will be reported using a code from Chapter 11: Diseases of the Digestive System, Chapter 13: Diseases of the Musculoskeletal System and Connective Tissue and Chapter 19: Injury, Poisoning and Certain Other Consequences of External

Causes. Codes from nearly all sections (A00–Z99) are also included so that findings arising from oral evaluations (e.g., "Z" codes) and relevant clinical information can be captured in the patient's dental record and included on a claim when necessary.

ICD-10-CM codes most applicable to dentistry are listed in this section of the CDT manual. Outside this section's scope are CDT to ICD mappings and medical claim coding. Information on these topics is available in the *CDT Companion* and other offerings in the ADA Store.

Note: ICD code guidance herein will assist in selection of appropriate diagnosis codes when a claim for dental services is being filed with the patient's medical benefit plan. Such claims can accommodate up to 12 ICD codes, and reporting requirements are more rigorous than what apply today for claims against dental benefit plans.

Information about the 1500 Health Insurance Claim Form used for claims filed against a patient's medical benefit plan is available online at *www.nucc.org/index.php/1500-claim-form-mainmenu-35.*

ICD code capture is addressed on page 32 of the "1500" form completion instructions.

Introduction

ICD-10-CM codes listed in the following chapters are extracted from the tabular list published by the Centers for Medicare and Medicaid Services (CMS) available online at *www.cms.gov/Medicare/Coding/ICD10*.

CMS also publishes general information on an ICD code's format and how they are reported on a claim submission. This information, in summary form, follows.

Note: The ICD-10-CM coding information in this section is at an introductory level. It is intended to familiarize dentists and practice staff with the code set and prompt its use to record diagnostic and descriptive information on patient records and dental claims.

More specific usage information as ICD-10-CM implementation continues will be contained in future editions. For now, such usage information is found in the Tabular List published by CMS, referenced above.

ICD Code Format

The ICD-10-CM Tabular List contains categories, subcategories, and codes, which are combinations of letters, numbers, or both.

- All categories are 3 characters, and a three-character category that has no further subdivision is equivalent to a code.

- Subcategories are either 4 or 5 characters.

- Codes may be 3, 4, 5, 6, or 7 characters; the decimal point is not included in the character count.

- Only complete codes are permissible for reporting, and any applicable 7th character must be assigned.

- Some codes have a placeholder character "X" that is designated for future expansion.

- Some codes have a character that must always be the 7th character in the data field. Codes that have a mandatory 7th character, but not always a 4th, 5th or 6th character, the placeholder "X" must be entered to fill any empty character spaces – e.g., K02.XXX7. An example of a 7th character code with a placeholder "X" would be the initial evaluation of a traumatic fracture of the right upper central incisor S02.5XXA.

General ICD Coding Concepts

An accurate diagnosis, appropriately coded, enables preparation of a treatment plan for necessary dental care that addresses the disease processes and related conditions identified by the dentist.

There are guidelines that a dentist should be aware of when documenting ICD codes in a patient record and on a claim.

1. The first ICD code listed on a patient's dental record and claim for procedures delivered on a specific date of service should be the primary reason for services provided during the office visit.

   a. The second through fourth ICD codes listed are the additional diagnoses applicable to the services provided during the visit.

   b. All ICD codes must clearly document the patient's condition and clinically support the planned and delivered treatment.

   c. Diagnosis information contributes to a robust patient record that supports the dentist's clinical decisions should there be a post-delivery review.

2. Each unique ICD-10-CM diagnosis code may be reported only once for an encounter.

3. An examination with abnormal findings refers to a condition or diagnosis that is newly identified or a change in severity of a chronic condition (e.g., periodontitis) during a routine oral examination.

   a. When assigning a code for "with abnormal findings," additional code(s) should be assigned to identify the specific abnormal finding(s).

4. "Z" codes allow for the description of encounters for routine or preventive examinations; they are not used if the examination is for diagnosis of a suspected condition or for treatment purposes. In such cases, the diagnosis code is used.

Helpful Hints for ICD-10-CM Coding

Per ICD-10-CM Guidelines, to assign a diagnosis code, the condition has to impact the patient care. "Code all documented conditions that coexist at the time of the encounter/visit and require or affect patient care treatment or management. Do not code conditions that were previously treated and no longer exist. However, history codes (categories Z80–Z87) may be used as secondary codes if the historical condition or family history has an impact on current care or influences treatment."

Users will notice coding guidance within the index and tabular section of ICD-10-CM. Some of this information is noted below and will assist the user in assigning the correct diagnosis code.

"Other" Codes – Codes titled "other" or "other specified" are for use when the information in the patient record provides detail for which a specific code does not exist. Alphabetic index entries with NEC (Not Elsewhere Classified) in the line designate "other" codes in the tabular list. These alphabetic index entries represent specific disease entities for which no specific code exists so the term is included within an "other" code.

"Unspecified" Codes – Codes titled "unspecified" are for use when the information in the patient record is insufficient to assign a more specific code. For those categories for which an unspecified code is not provided, the "other specified" code may represent both other and unspecified.

Inclusion Terms Note – An "inclusion terms note" is a list of terms included under some codes. These terms are the conditions for which that code is to be used. The terms may be synonyms of the code title, or, in the case of "other specified codes," the terms are a list of the various conditions assigned to that code. The inclusion terms are not necessarily exhaustive. Additional terms found in the Alphabetical Index may also be assigned to a code.

"Code Also" Note – A "code also" note instructs that two codes may be required to fully describe a condition, but this note does not provide sequencing direction. The sequencing depends on the circumstances of the encounter.

"Use Additional Code" Notes – "Use additional code" notes are found in the Tabular List at codes that are not part of an etiology/manifestation pair where a secondary code is useful to fully describe a condition. The sequencing rule is the same as the etiology/manifestation pair, "use additional code" indicates that a secondary code should be added, if known.

Sequela (Late Effects) – A sequela is the residual effect (condition produced) after the acute phase of an illness or injury has terminated. There is no time limit on when a sequela code can be used.

A Note about the Use of Mental Health and Substance Abuse Codes

While several mental health and substance abuse codes have been included in the list below, please assign those diagnoses with care. ICD-10-CM codes related to mental health conditions, substance abuse, or Human Immunodeficiency Virus (HIV) are protected by the Health Insurance Portability and Accountability Act (HIPAA). Individual state laws may supersede HIPAA when they are more stringent than the federal rules.

Select ICD-10-CM Codes Applicable to Dentistry

Presentation Format:

ICD-10-CM codes and their meanings are presented in 21 separate sections, as seen in this section's Table of Contents. Each of these sections can have one or more chapters where individual ICD codes are listed in ascending alphanumerical order. These sections and chapters reflect the various types of patient encounters and clinical conditions (current and past) that would be considered when treatment planning.

1. Dental Encounters

Examinations

Z01.20	Encounter for dental examination and cleaning without abnormal findings
Z01.21	Encounter for dental examination and cleaning with abnormal findings
Z01.812	Encounter for other preprocedural laboratory examinations
Z01.818	Encounter for other preprocedural examinations
Z01.89	Encounter for other specified special examinations
Z02.6	Encounter for examination for insurance purposes
Z04.1	Encounter for examination and observation following transport accident
Z04.2	Encounter for examination and observation following work accident
Z04.3	Encounter for examination and observation following other accident
Z04.89	Encounter for examination and observation for other specified reasons
Z04.9	Encounter for examination and observation for unspecified reason
Z08	Encounter for follow-up examination after completed treatment for malignant neoplasm
Z09	Encounter for follow-up examination after completed treatment for conditions other than malignant neoplasm
Z12.81	Encounter for screening for malignant neoplasm or oral cavity
Z13.84	Encounter for screening for dental disorders
Z33.1	Pregnant state, incidental
Z41.1	Encounter for cosmetic surgery
Z48.814	Encounter for the surgical aftercare following surgery on the teeth or oral cavity

Preventive Care

Z29.3	Encounter for prophylactic fluoride administration
Z29.81	Encounter for HIV pre-exposure prophylaxis
Z29.89	Encounter for other specified prophylactic measures
Z29.9	Encounter for prophylactic measures, unspecified
Z71.3	Dietary counselling and surveillance
Z71.41	Alcohol counselling and surveillance of alcoholic
Z71.51	Drug abuse counselling and surveillance of drug abuser
Z71.6	Tobacco use and counselling

Post-procedure Complications (Aftercare)

M27.51	Perforation of root canal space due to endodontic treatment
M27.52	Endodontic overfill
M27.59	Other periradicular pathology associated with previous endodontic treatment
T86.820	Skin graft (allograft) rejection
T86.821	Skin graft (allograft) (autograft) failure
T86.822	Skin graft (allograft) (autograft) infection — Use additional code to specify infection
T86.828	Other complications of skin graft (allograft) (autograft)
T86.830	Bone graft rejection
T86.831	Bone graft failure
T86.832	Bone graft infection — Use additional code to specify infection
T86.838	Other complications of bone graft

Post-procedural Aftercare

Z46.3	Encounter for fitting and adjustment of dental prosthetic device
Z46.4	Encounter for fitting and adjustment of orthodontic device
Z48.00	Encounter for change or removal of nonsurgical wound dressing
Z48.01	Encounter for change or removal of surgical wound dressing
Z48.02	Encounter for removal of sutures
Z48.03	Encounter for change or removal of drains
Z48.1	Encounter for planned postprocedural wound closure
Z48.3	Aftercare following surgery for neoplasm

Z48.814	Encounter for surgical aftercare following surgery on the teeth or oral cavity
Z48.89	Encounter for other specified surgical aftercare
Z51.5	Encounter for palliative care
Z51.89	Encounter for other specified aftercare
Z71.2	Person consulting for explanation of examination or test findings

Procedures or Treatment Not Carried Out

Z53.01	Procedure and treatment not carried out due to patient smoking
Z53.09	Procedure and treatment not carried out because of other contraindication
Z53.1	Procedure and treatment not carried out because of patient's decision for reasons of belief and group pressure
Z53.20	Procedure and treatment not carried out because of patient's decision for unspecified reasons
Z53.21	Procedure and treatment not carried out due to patient leaving prior to being seen by health care provider
Z53.29	Procedure and treatment not carried out because of patient's decision for other reasons
Z53.9	Procedure and treatment not carried out, unspecified reason

2. Dental Caries

Risk Factors

Z91.841	Risk for dental caries, low
Z91.842	Risk for dental caries, moderate
Z91.843	Risk for dental caries, high

Caries

K02.3	Arrested dental caries (decay and cavities) (includes coronal and root caries)
K02.51	Dental caries on pit and fissure surface limited to enamel
K02.52	Dental caries on pit and fissure surface penetrating into dentin
K02.53	Dental caries on pit and fissure surface penetrating into pulp
K02.61	Dental caries on smooth surface limited to enamel
K02.62	Dental caries on smooth surface penetrating into dentin
K02.63	Dental caries on smooth surface penetrating into pulp
K02.7	Dental root caries
K02.9	Dental caries, unspecified

3. Disorders of Teeth

Occlusal Trauma

K08.81   Primary occlusal trauma

K08.82   Secondary occlusal trauma

K08.89   Other specified disorders of teeth and supporting structures
(Includes the following — Enlargement of alveolar ridge NOS [not
otherwise specified]; Insufficient anatomic crown height, Insufficient
clinical crown length; Irregular alveolar process; Toothache NOS)

Tooth Wear

K03.0   Excessive attrition of teeth

K03.1   Abrasion of teeth

K03.2   Erosion of teeth

K03.3   Pathological resorption of teeth

Other Disorders

K03.4   Hypercementosis

K03.5   Ankylosis of teeth

K03.6   Deposits [accretions] on teeth

K03.7   Posteruptive color changes of dental hard tissues

K03.81   Cracked tooth

K03.89   Other specified diseases of hard tissues of teeth

K03.9   Disease of hard tissues of teeth, unspecified

4. Disorders of Pulp and Periapical Tissues

K04.01   Reversible pulpitis

K04.02   Irreversible pulpitis

K04.1   Necrosis of pulp

K04.2   Pulp degeneration

K04.3   Abnormal hard tissue formation in pulp

K04.4   Acute apical periodontitis of pulpal origin

K04.5   Chronic apical periodontitis

K04.6   Periapical abscess with sinus

K04.7   Periapical abscess without sinus

K04.8   Radicular cyst

K04.99   Other diseases of pulp and periapical tissues

5. Diseases and Conditions of the Periodontium

Gingivitis

K05.00   Acute gingivitis, plaque induced

K05.01   Acute gingivitis, non-plaque induced

K05.10   Chronic gingivitis, plaque induced

K05.11   Chronic gingivitis, non-plaque induced

Gingival Recession

K06.011 Localized gingival recession, minimal

K06.012 Localized gingival recession, moderate

K06.013 Localized gingival recession, severe

K06.021 Generalized gingival recession, minimal

K06.022 Generalized gingival recession, moderate

K06.023 Generalized gingival recession, severe

Other Gingival Conditions

K06.1   Gingival enlargement

K06.2   Gingival and edentulous alveolar ridge lesions associated with trauma

K06.3   Horizontal alveolar bone loss

K06.8   Other specified disorders of gingiva and edentulous alveolar ridge

Periodontitis

K05.211 Aggressive periodontitis, localized, slight

K05.212 Aggressive periodontitis, localized, moderate

K05.213 Aggressive periodontitis, localized, severe

K05.221 Aggressive periodontitis, generalized, slight

K05.222 Aggressive periodontitis, generalized, moderate

K05.223 Aggressive periodontitis, generalized, severe

K05.311 Chronic periodontitis, localized, slight

K05.312   Chronic periodontitis, localized, moderate

K05.313   Chronic periodontitis, localized, severe

K05.321   Chronic periodontitis, generalized, slight

K05.322   Chronic periodontitis, generalized, moderate

K05.323   Chronic periodontitis, generalized, severe

K05.4   Periodontosis

K05.5   Other periodontal disease

6. Alveolar Ridge Disorders

Atrophy of Alveolar Ridge

K08.21   Minimal atrophy of the mandible

K08.22   Moderate atrophy of the mandible

K08.23   Severe atrophy of the mandible

K08.24   Minimal atrophy of maxilla

K08.25   Moderate atrophy of the maxilla

K08.26   Severe atrophy of the maxilla

Alveolar Anomalies

M26.71   Alveolar maxillary hyperplasia

M26.72   Alveolar mandibular hyperplasia

M26.73   Alveolar maxillary hypoplasia

M26.74   Alveolar mandibular hypoplasia

M26.79   Other specified alveolar anomalies

7. Findings of Lost Teeth

Class I: stage of edentulism that is most apt to be successfully treated with complete dentures using conventional prosthodontic techniques.

Class II: characterized by the continued physical degradation of the denture-supporting anatomy. It is also characterized by the early onset of systemic disease interactions and by specific patient management and lifestyle considerations.

Class III: characterized by the need for surgical revision of supporting structures to allow for adequate prosthodontic function.

Class IV: the most debilitating requiring reconstructive surgery when all teeth are missing or the most severely compromised oral manifestations with poor outcome prognosis in partial edentulism. Treatment is primarily prosthodontic in nature with missing teeth or adjacent structures being restored or replaced with artificial, biocompatible structures.

Lost Teeth: Unspecified Causes

K08.101	Complete loss of teeth, unspecified cause, class I
K08.102	Complete loss of teeth, unspecified cause, class II
K08.103	Complete loss of teeth, unspecified cause, class III
K08.104	Complete loss of teeth, unspecified cause, class IV
K08.401	Partial loss of teeth, unspecified cause, class I
K08.402	Partial loss of teeth, unspecified cause, class II
K08.403	Partial loss of teeth, unspecified cause, class III
K08.404	Partial loss of teeth, unspecified cause, class IV

Lost Teeth: Specified Causes

K08.0	Exfoliation of teeth due to systemic causes
K08.191	Complete loss of teeth due to other specified cause, class I
K08.192	Complete loss of teeth due to other specified cause, class II
K08.193	Complete loss of teeth due to other specified cause, class III
K08.194	Complete loss of teeth due to other specified cause, class IV
K08.491	Partial loss of teeth due to other specified cause, class I
K08.492	Partial loss of teeth due to other specified cause, class II
K08.493	Partial loss of teeth due to other specified cause, class III
K08.494	Partial loss of teeth due to other specified cause, class IV

Lost Teeth: Trauma Related

K08.111	Complete loss of teeth due to trauma, class I
K08.112	Complete loss of teeth due to trauma, class II
K08.113	Complete loss of teeth due to trauma, class III
K08.114	Complete loss of teeth due to trauma, class IV
K08.411	Partial loss of teeth due to trauma, class I
K08.412	Partial loss of teeth due to trauma, class II
K08.413	Partial loss of teeth due to trauma, class III
K08.414	Partial loss of teeth due to trauma, class IV

Lost Teeth: Periodontitis Related

K08.121	Complete loss of teeth due to periodontal diseases, class I
K08.122	Complete loss of teeth due to periodontal diseases, class II
K08.123	Complete loss of teeth due to periodontal diseases, class III
K08.124	Complete loss of teeth due to periodontal diseases, class IV
K08.421	Partial loss of teeth due to periodontal diseases, class I
K08.422	Partial loss of teeth due to periodontal diseases, class II
K08.423	Partial loss of teeth due to periodontal diseases, class III
K08.424	Partial loss of teeth due to periodontal diseases, class IV

Lost Teeth: Caries Related

K08.131	Complete loss of teeth due to caries, class I
K08.132	Complete loss of teeth due to caries, class II
K08.133	Complete loss of teeth due to caries, class III
K08.134	Complete loss of teeth due to caries, class IV
K08.431	Partial loss of teeth due to caries, class I
K08.432	Partial loss of teeth due to caries, class II
K08.433	Partial loss of teeth due to caries, class III
K08.434	Partial loss of teeth due to caries, class IV

8. Developmental Disorders of Teeth and Jaws

Number of Teeth

K00.0	Anodontia
K00.1	Supernumerary teeth

Size and Form of Teeth

K00.2	Abnormalities of size and form of teeth
K00.3	Mottled teeth
K00.4	Disturbances in tooth formation
K00.5	Hereditary disturbances in tooth structure, not elsewhere classified
K00.8	Other disorders of tooth development

Tooth Eruption

K00.6	Disturbances in tooth eruption
K00.7	Teething syndrome
K01.0	Embedded teeth
K01.1	Impacted teeth
K08.3	Retained dental root
Z18.32	Retained tooth

Malocclusion

M26.211	Malocclusion, Angle's class I
M26.212	Malocclusion, Angle's class II
M26.213	Malocclusion, Angle's class III
M26.220	Open anterior occlusal relationship
M26.221	Open posterior occlusal relationship
M26.23	Excessive horizontal overlap
M26.24	Reverse articulation
M26.25	Anomalies of interarch distance
M26.29	Other anomalies of dental arch relationship
M26.30	Unspecified anomaly of tooth position of fully erupted tooth or teeth
M26.31	Crowding of fully erupted teeth
M26.32	Excessive spacing of fully erupted teeth
M26.33	Horizontal displacement of fully erupted tooth or teeth

M26.34   Vertical displacement of fully erupted tooth or teeth

M26.35   Rotation of fully erupted tooth or teeth

M26.36   Insufficient interocclusal distance of fully erupted teeth (ridge)

M26.37   Excessive interocclusal distance of fully erupted teeth

M26.39   Other anomalies of tooth position of fully erupted tooth or teeth

M26.51   Abnormal jaw closure

M26.52   Limited mandibular range of motion

M26.53   Deviation in opening and closing of the mandible

M26.54   Insufficient anterior guidance

M26.55   Centric occlusion maximum intercuspation discrepancy

M26.56   Non-working side interference

M26.57   Lack of posterior occlusal support

M26.59   Other dentofacial functional abnormalities

Jaw Anomalies

M26.01   Maxillary hyperplasia

M26.02   Maxillary hypoplasia

M26.03   Mandibular hyperplasia

M26.04   Mandibular hypoplasia

M26.05   Macrogenia

M26.06   Microgenia

M26.07   Excessive tuberosity of jaw

M26.10   Unspecified anomaly of jaw-cranial base relationship

M26.11   Maxillary asymmetry

M26.12   Other jaw asymmetry

M26.19   Other specified anomalies of jaw-cranial base relationship

M26.20   Unspecified anomaly of dental arch relationship

Other Dentofacial Anomalies

M26.81   Anterior soft tissue impingement

M26.82   Posterior soft tissue impingement

M26.89   Other dentofacial anomalies

Cleft Lip and Palate

Q35.1	Cleft hard palate
Q35.3	Cleft soft palate
Q35.5	Cleft hard palate with cleft soft palate
Q35.7	Cleft uvula
Q36.0	Cleft lip, bilateral
Q36.1	Cleft lip, median
Q36.9	Cleft lip, unilateral
Q37.0	Cleft hard palate with bilateral cleft lip
Q37.1	Cleft hard palate with unilateral cleft lip
Q37.2	Cleft soft palate with bilateral cleft lip
Q37.3	Cleft soft palate with unilateral cleft lip
Q37.4	Cleft hard and soft palate with bilateral cleft lip
Q37.5	Cleft hard and soft palate with unilateral cleft lip

Congenital Malformations of Mouth, Tongue and Pharynx

Q38.0	Congenital malformations of lips, not elsewhere classified
Q38.1	Ankyloglossia
Q38.2	Macroglossia
Q38.3	Other congenital malformations of tongue
Q38.4	Congenital malformations of salivary glands and ducts
Q38.5	Congenital malformations of palate, not elsewhere classified
Q38.6	Other congenital malformations of mouth

9. Treatment Complications

Endodontic Complications

M27.51	Perforation of root canal space due to endodontic treatment
M27.52	Endodontic overfill
M27.53	Endodontic underfill
M27.59	Other periradicular pathology associated with previous endodontic treatment

Implant Failure

M27.61   Osseointegration failure of dental implant

M27.62   Post-osseointegration biological failure of dental implant

M27.63   Post-osseointegration mechanical failure of dental implant

M27.69   Other endosseous dental implant failure

Unsatisfactory Restorations

K08.51   Open restoration margins of tooth

K08.52   Unrepairable overhanging of dental restorative materials

K08.530   Fractured dental restorative material without loss of material

K08.531   Fractured dental restorative material with loss of material

K08.54   Contour of existing restoration of tooth biologically incompatible with oral health

K08.55   Allergy to existing dental restorative material

K08.56   Poor aesthetic of existing restoration of tooth

K08.59   Other unsatisfactory restoration of tooth

Complications of Surgical and Medical Care

Note: The appropriate 7th character is to be added to each code that displays an asterisk (*) in the section Complications of Surgical and Medical Care. Insert an "X" as needed as placeholder for unused spaces (e.g., T81.83XA; T81.83XD; T81.83XS).
   A = Initial encounter
   D = Subsequent encounter
   S = Sequela

T81.83X*   Persistent postprocedural fistula

T84.318   Breakdown (mechanical) of other bone devices, implants and grafts

T84.328   Displacement of other bone devices, implants and grafts

T84.398   Other mechanical complication of other bone devices, implants and grafts

T84.59X*   Infection and inflammatory reaction due to other internal joint prosthesis

T85.79X*   Infection and inflammatory reaction due to other internal prosthetic devices, implants and grafts

T88.52X*   Failed moderate sedation during procedure

T88.53X*   Unintended awareness under general anesthesia during procedure

T88.59X*   Other complications of anesthesia

T88.6XX*	Anaphylactic reaction due to adverse effect of correct drug or medicament properly administered
T88.7	Unspecified adverse effect of drug or medicament
T88.8XX*	Other specified complications of surgical and medical care, not elsewhere classified
T88.9	Complication of surgical and medical care, unspecified

Other Post-procedural States

Z98.810	Dental sealant status
Z98.811	Dental restoration status
Z98.818	Other dental procedure status

10. Inflammatory Conditions of the Mucosa

Stomatitis

K12.0	Recurrent oral aphthae
K12.1	Other forms of stomatitis
K12.2	Cellulitis and abscess of mouth
K12.31	Oral mucositis (ulcerative) due to antineoplastic therapy
K12.32	Oral mucositis (ulcerative) due to other drugs
K12.33	Oral mucositis (ulcerative) due to radiation
K12.39	Other oral mucositis (ulcerative)

11. TMJ Diseases and Conditions

TMJ Disorders

M26.601	Right temporomandibular joint disorder, unspecified
M26.602	Left temporomandibular joint disorder, unspecified
M26.603	Bilateral temporomandibular joint disorder, unspecified
M26.609	Unspecified temporomandibular joint disorder, unspecified side
M26.69	Other specified disorders of temporomandibular joint

Adhesions and Ankylosis

| M26.611 | Adhesions and ankylosis of right temporomandibular joint |
| M26.612 | Adhesions and ankylosis of left temporomandibular joint |

M26.613   Adhesions and ankylosis of bilateral temporomandibular joint

Arthralgia

M26.621   Arthralgia of right temporomandibular joint

M26.622   Arthralgia of left temporomandibular joint

M26.623   Arthralgia of bilateral temporomandibular joint

Aricular Disc Disorders

M26.631   Articular disc disorder of right temporomandibular joint

M26.632   Articular disc disorder of left temporomandibular joint

M26.633   Articular disc disorder of bilateral temporomandibular joint

Arthritis of Temporomandibular Joint

M26.641   Arthritis of right temporomandibular joint

M26.642   Arthritis of left temporomandibular joint

M26.643   Arthritis of bilateral temporomandibular joint

Arthropathy of Temporomandibular Joint

M26.651   Arthropathy of right temporomandibular joint

M26.652   Arthropathy of left temporomandibular joint

M26.653   Arthropathy of bilateral temporomandibular joint

12. Breathing, Speech and Sleep Disorders

Mouthbreathing

R06.5   Mouth breathing

R06.83   Snoring

R06.89   Other abnormalities of breathing

Speech

R47.9   Unspecified speech disturbances

F80.89   Other developmental disorders of speech and language

F80.9   Developmental disorder of speech and language, unspecified

Sleep Related Breathing Disorders

G47.30   Sleep apnea, unspecified

G47.31   Primary central sleep apnea

G47.32   High altitude periodic breathing

G47.33   Obstructive sleep apnea (adult) (pediatric)

G47.34   Idiopathic sleep related nonobstructive alveolar hypoventilation

G47.35   Congenital central alveolar hypoventilation syndrome

G47.36   Sleep related hypoventilation in conditions classified elsewhere

G47.37   Central sleep apnea in conditions classified elsewhere

G47.39   Other sleep apnea

G47.63   Sleep related bruxism

G47.8   Other sleep disorders

G47.9   Sleep disorder, unspecified

13. Trauma and Related Conditions

Soft Tissue Injuries

Note: The appropriate 7th character is to be added to each code in this chapter (Soft Tissue Injuries). Insert an "X" as needed as placeholder for unused spaces (e.g., S00.511A; S00.0511D; S00.0511S).

- A = Initial encounter
- D = Subsequent encounter
- S = Sequela

S00.511   Abrasion of lip

S00.512   Abrasion of oral cavity

S00.521   Blister (nonthermal) of lip

S00.522   Blister (nonthermal) of oral cavity

S00.531   Contusion of lip

S00.532   Contusion of oral cavity

S00.541   External constriction of lip

S00.542   External constriction of oral cavity

S01.511   Laceration without foreign body of lip

S01.512   Laceration without foreign body of oral cavity

S01.521   Laceration with foreign body of lip

S01.522   Laceration with foreign body of oral cavity

S01.531   Puncture wound without foreign body of lip

S01.532   Puncture wound without foreign body of oral cavity

S01.541   Puncture wound with foreign body of lip

S01.542   Puncture wound with foreign body of oral cavity

S01.551   Open bite of lip

S01.552   Open bite of oral cavity

Dislocation of Jaw

Note: The appropriate 7th character is to be added to each code in this chapter (Dislocation of Jaw). Insert an "X" as needed as placeholder for unused spaces (e.g., S03.00XA; S03.00XD; S03.00XS).

- A = Initial encounter
- D = Subsequent encounter
- S = Sequela

S03.01X* Dislocation of jaw, right side

S03.02X* Dislocation of jaw, left side

S03.03X* Dislocation of jaw, bilateral

S03.2XX* Dislocation of tooth

S03.41X* Sprain of jaw, right side

S03.42X* Sprain of jaw, left side

S03.43X* Sprain of jaw, bilateral

Fractures: Nasal Bones

Note: The appropriate 7th character is to be added to each code for all "Fractures" which include Nasal bones through Skull and Facial bones. These codes are found in Chapter 19 Injury, Poisoning and Certain Other Consequences of External Causes. Insert an "X" as needed as placeholder for unused spaces (e.g., S02.2XXA; S02.2XXB; S02.2XXD; S02.2XXG; S02.2XXK; S02.2XXS).

- A = initial encounter for closed fracture
- B = initial encounter for open fracture
- D = subsequent encounter for fracture with routine healing
- G = subsequent encounter for fracture with delayed healing
- K = subsequent encounter for fracture with nonunion
- S = sequela

S02.2XX* Fracture of nasal bones

Fractures: Malar

S02.40A Malar fracture, right side

S02.40B Malar fracture, left side

Fractures: Maxilla

S02.40C Maxillary fracture, right side

S02.40D Maxillary fracture, left side

Fractures: Zygoma

S02.40E   Zygomatic fracture, right side

S02.40F   Zygomatic fracture, left side

Fractures: LeFort

S02.411   LeFort I fracture

S02.412   LeFort II fracture

S02.413   LeFort III fracture

Tooth Fractures

S02.5XX*   Fracture of tooth (traumatic)

Fractures: Mandible

S02.601   Fracture of unspecified part of body of right mandible

S02.602   Fracture of unspecified part of body of left mandible

S02.611   Fracture of condylar process of right mandible

S02.612   Fracture of condylar process of left mandible

S02.621   Fracture of subcondylar process of right mandible

S02.622   Fracture of subcondylar process of left mandible

S02.631   Fracture of coronoid process of right mandible

S02.632   Fracture of coronoid process of left mandible

S02.641   Fracture of ramus of right mandible

S02.642   Fracture of ramus of left mandible

S02.651   Fracture of angle of right mandible

S02.652   Fracture of angle of left mandible

S02.66X*   Fracture of symphysis of mandible

S02.69X*   Fracture of mandible of other specified site

Alveolar Fractures

S02.42X*   Fracture of alveolus of maxilla

S02.671   Fracture of alveolus of right mandible

S02.672   Fracture of alveolus of left mandible

Fractures: Skull and Facial Bones

S02.81X*   Fracture of other specified skull and facial bones, right side

S02.82X*   Fracture of other specified skull and facial bones, left side

S02.91   Unspecified fracture of skull

S02.92   Unspecified fracture of facial bones

Foreign Bodies

Note: The appropriate 7th character is to be added to each code in this chapter (Foreign Bodies). Insert an "X" as needed as placeholder for unused spaces (e.g., T17.0XXA; T17.0XXD; T17.0XXS).
    A = Initial encounter
    D = Subsequent encounter
    S = Sequela

T17.0XX*   Foreign body in nasal sinus

S00.551   Superficial foreign body of lip

S00.552   Superficial foreign body of oral cavity

S01.521   Laceration with foreign body of lip

S01.522   Laceration with foreign body of oral cavity

S01.541   Puncture wound with foreign body of lip

S01.542   Puncture wound with foreign body of oral cavity

14. Oral Neoplasms

Malignant: Lip

C00.0   Malignant neoplasm of external upper lip

C00.1   Malignant neoplasm of external lower lip

C00.2   Malignant neoplasm of external lip, unspecified

C00.3   Malignant neoplasm of upper lip, inner aspect

C00.4   Malignant neoplasm of lower lip, inner aspect

C00.5   Malignant neoplasm of lip, unspecified, inner aspect

C00.6   Malignant neoplasm of commissure of lip, unspecified

C00.8   Malignant neoplasm of overlapping sites of lip

C00.9   Malignant neoplasm of lip, unspecified

C44.01   Basal cell carcinoma of skin of lip

C44.02   Squamous cell carcinoma of skin of lip

C44.09   Other specified malignant neoplasm of skin of lip

Malignant: Tongue

C01   Malignant neoplasm of base of tongue

C02.0   Malignant neoplasm of dorsal surface of tongue

C02.1   Malignant neoplasm of border of tongue

C02.2   Malignant neoplasm of ventral surface of tongue

C02.3   Malignant neoplasm of anterior two-thirds of tongue, part unspecified

C02.8   Malignant neoplasm of overlapping sites of tongue

Malignant: Gums

C03.0   Malignant neoplasm of upper gum

C03.1   Malignant neoplasm of lower gum

C03.9   Malignant neoplasm of gum, unspecified

Malignant: Floor of the Mouth

C04.0   Malignant neoplasm of anterior floor of mouth

C04.1   Malignant neoplasm of lateral floor of mouth

C04.8   Malignant neoplasm of overlapping sites of floor of mouth

C04.9   Malignant neoplasm of floor of mouth, unspecified

Malignant: Palate

C05.0   Malignant neoplasm of hard palate

C05.1   Malignant neoplasm of soft palate

C05.8   Malignant neoplasm of overlapping sites of palate

C05.9   Malignant neoplasm of palate, unspecified

Malignant: Oropharyngeal Region

C05.2   Malignant neoplasm of uvula

C02.4   Malignant neoplasm of lingual tonsil

C09.0   Malignant neoplasm of tonsillar fossa

C09.1   Malignant neoplasm of tonsillar pillar (anterior) (posterior)

C09.8   Malignant neoplasm of overlapping sites of tonsil

C09.9   Malignant neoplasm of tonsil, unspecified

C10.0   Malignant neoplasm of vallecula

C10.1   Malignant neoplasm of anterior surface of epiglottis

C10.2   Malignant neoplasm of lateral wall of oropharynx

C10.3   Malignant neoplasm of posterior wall of oropharynx

C10.4   Malignant neoplasm of branchial cleft

C10.8   Malignant neoplasm of overlapping sites of oropharynx

C10.9   Malignant neoplasm of oropharynx, unspecified

Malignant: Other Areas

C06.0   Malignant neoplasm of cheek mucosa

C06.1   Malignant neoplasm of vestibule of mouth

C06.2   Malignant neoplasm of retromolar area

C06.80 Malignant neoplasm of overlapping sites of unspecified parts of mouth

C06.89 Malignant neoplasm of overlapping sites of other parts of mouth

C06.9   Malignant neoplasm of mouth, unspecified

C41.0   Malignant neoplasm of bones of skull and face

C41.1   Malignant neoplasm of mandible

C76.0   Malignant neoplasm of head, face and neck

Malignant: Salivary Glands

C07   Malignant neoplasm of parotid gland

C08.0   Malignant neoplasm of submandibular gland

C08.1   Malignant neoplasm of sublingual gland

C08.9   Malignant neoplasm of major salivary gland, unspecified

Carcinoma in Situ

D00.00 Carcinoma in situ of oral cavity, unspecified site

D00.01 Carcinoma in situ of labial mucosa and vermilion border

D00.02 Carcinoma in situ of buccal mucosa

D00.03 Carcinoma in situ of gingiva and edentulous alveolar ridge

D00.04 Carcinoma in situ of soft palate

D00.05 Carcinoma in situ of hard palate

D00.06 Carcinoma in situ of floor of mouth

D00.07 Carcinoma in situ of tongue

D00.08 Carcinoma in situ of pharynx

D04.0   Carcinoma in situ of skin of lip

Benign Neoplasms

D10.0	Benign neoplasm of lip
D10.1	Benign neoplasm of tongue
D10.2	Benign neoplasm of floor of mouth
D10.30	Benign neoplasm of unspecified part of mouth
D10.39	Benign neoplasm of other parts of mouth
D10.4	Benign neoplasm of tonsil
D10.5	Benign neoplasm of other parts of oropharynx

15. Pathologies

Jaw Related

M27.0	Developmental disorders of jaws
M27.1	Giant cell granuloma, central
M27.2	Inflammatory conditions of jaws
M27.3	Alveolitis of jaws
M27.40	Unspecified cyst of jaw
M27.49	Other cysts of jaw
M27.8	Other specified diseases of jaws

Cysts

K09.0	Developmental odontogenic cysts
K09.1	Developmental (nonodontogenic) cysts of oral region
K09.8	Other cysts of oral region, not elsewhere classified

Salivary Glands

K11.0	Atrophy of salivary gland
K11.1	Hypertrophy of salivary gland
K11.21	Acute sialoadenitis
K11.22	Acute recurrent sialoadenitis
K11.23	Chronic sialoadenitis
K11.3	Abscess of salivary gland
K11.4	Fistula of salivary gland
K11.5	Sialolithiasis
K11.6	Mucocele of salivary gland

K11.7	Disturbances of salivary secretion
K11.8	Other diseases of salivary glands

Lips and Oral Mucosa

K13.1	Cheek and lip biting
K13.21	Leukoplakia of oral mucosa, including tongue
K13.22	Minimal keratinized residual ridge mucosa
K13.23	Excessive keratinized residual ridge mucosa
K13.24	Leukokeratosis nicotina palate
K13.29	Other disturbances of oral epithelium, including tongue
K13.3	Hairy leukoplakia
K13.4	Granuloma and granuloma-like lesions of oral mucosa
K13.5	Oral submucous fibrosis
K13.6	Irritative hyperplasia of oral mucosa
K13.79	Other lesions of oral mucosa

Tongue

K14.0	Glossitis
K14.1	Geographic tongue
K14.2	Median rhomboid glossitis
K14.3	Hypertrophy of tongue papillae
K14.4	Atrophy of tongue papillae
K14.5	Plicated tongue
K14.6	Glossodynia
K14.8	Other diseases of tongue

Skin and Subcutaneous Tissues

L40.52	Psoriatric arthritis mutilans
L40.54	Psoriatic juvenile arthropathy
L40.59	Other psoriatic arthropathy
L43.9	Lichen planus, unspecified
L90.5	Scar conditions and fibrosis of skin

Musculoskeletal System and Connective Tissue

M06.9	Rheumatoid arthritis, unspecified

M08.00   Unspecified juvenile rheumatoid arthritis of unspecified site

M24.20   Disorder of ligament, unspecified site

M32.10   Systemic lupus erythematosus, organ or system involvement unspecified

M35.00   Sjögren syndrome [Sicca], unspecified

M35.0C   Sjögren syndrome with dental involvement

M35.7   Hypermobility syndrome

M43.6   Torticollis

M45.9   Ankylosing spondylitis of unspecified sites in spine

M54.2   Cervicalgia

M60.9   Myositis, unspecified

M62.40   Contracture of muscle, unspecified site

M62.81   Muscle weakness (generalized)

M62.838   Other muscle spasm

M65.9   Synovitis and tenosynovitis, unspecified

S00.511A   Abrasion of lip, initial encounter

S00.511D   Abrasion of lip, subsequent encounter

S00.511S   Abrasion of lip, sequela

M79.2   Neuralgia and neuritis, unspecified

M87.00   Idiopathic aseptic necrosis of unspecified bone

M87.180   Osteonecrosis due to drugs, jaw

16. Medical Findings Related to Dental Treatment

Communicable Diseases

A69.20   Lyme disease, unspecified

B00.0   Eczema herpeticum (Kaposi's varicelliform eruption)

B00.1   Herpesviral vesicular dermatitis

B00.2   Herpesviral gingivostomatitis and pharyngotonsillitis

B37.0   Candidal stomatitis (Oral Thrush)

U07.1   COVID-19

Diabetes

E08.630	Diabetes mellitus due to underlying condition with periodontal disease
E08.638	Diabetes mellitus due to underlying condition with other oral complications
E09.630	Drug or chemical induced diabetes mellitus with periodontal disease
E09.638	Drug or chemical induced diabetes mellitus with other oral complications
E10.630	Type 1 diabetes mellitus with periodontal disease
E10.638	Type 1 diabetes mellitus with other oral complications
E10.9	Type 1 diabetes mellitus without complications
E11.630	Type 2 diabetes mellitus with periodontal disease
E11.638	Type 2 diabetes mellitus with other oral complications
E11.9	Type 2 diabetes mellitus without complications
E13.630	Other specified diabetes mellitus with periodontal disease
E13.638	Other specified diabetes mellitus with other oral complications
R73.01	Impaired fasting glucose
R73.02	Impaired glucose tolerance (oral)
R73.03	Prediabetes
R73.09	Other abnormal glucose
R73.9	Hyperglycemia, unspecified

Substance Abuse/Tobacco Use

Z71.6	Tobacco abuse counseling
Z72.0	Tobacco use
F17.200	Nicotine dependence, unspecified, uncomplicated
F17.210	Nicotine dependence, cigarettes, uncomplicated
F17.220	Nicotine dependence, chewing tobacco, uncomplicated
F17.290	Nicotine dependence, other tobacco products, uncomplicated

New Diseases of Uncertain Etiology

U07.0	Vaping related disorder

Substance Abuse/Alcohol Use

F10.10	Alcohol abuse, uncomplicated
F10.11	Alcohol abuse, in remission
F10.129	Alcohol abuse with intoxication, unspecified
F10.19	Alcohol abuse with unspecified alcohol-induced disorder

Family History

Z80.0	Family history of malignant neoplasm of digestive organs
Z81.0	Family history of intellectual disabilities
Z81.1	Family history of alcohol abuse and dependence
Z81.2	Family history of tobacco abuse and dependence
Z81.3	Family history of other psychoactive substance abuse and dependence
Z81.4	Family history of other substance abuse and dependence
Z81.8	Family history of other mental and behavioral disorders
Z83.0	Family history of human immunodeficiency virus [HIV] disease
Z83.2	Family history of diseases of the blood and blood-forming organs and certain disorders involving the immune mechanism
Z83.3	Family history of diabetes mellitus
Z83.49	Family history of other endocrine, nutritional and metabolic diseases
Z83.79	Family history of other diseases of the digestive system

Personal History

F41.9	Anxiety disorder, unspecified
R45.0	Nervousness
P92.9	Feeding problem of newborn, unspecified
Z85.00	Personal history of malignant neoplasm of unspecified digestive organ
Z85.810	Personal history of malignant neoplasm of tongue
Z85.818	Personal history of malignant neoplasm of other sites of lip, oral cavity, and pharynx
Z85.819	Personal history of malignant neoplasm of unspecified site of lip, oral cavity, and pharynx
Z85.830	Personal history of malignant neoplasm of bone
Z85.831	Personal history of malignant neoplasm of soft tissue
Z86.003	Personal history of in-situ neoplasm of oral cavity, esophagus and stomach
Z87.730	Personal history (corrected) of cleft lip and palate

Z87.738	Personal history of other specified (corrected) congenital malformations of digestive system
Z88.0	Allergy status to penicillin
Z88.1	Allergy status to other antibiotic agents status
Z88.2	Allergy status to sulfonamides status
Z88.3	Allergy status to other anti-infective agents status
Z88.4	Allergy status to anesthetic agent status
Z88.5	Allergy status to narcotic agent status
Z88.6	Allergy status to analgesic agent status
Z88.7	Allergy status to serum and vaccine status
Z88.8	Allergy status to other drugs, medicaments and biological substances status
Z88.9	Allergy status to unspecified drugs, medicaments and biological substances status
Z91.09	Other allergy status, other than to drugs and biological substances
Z91.19	Patient's noncompliance with other medical treatment and regimen
Z91.190	Patient's noncompliance with other medical treatment and regimen due to financial hardship
Z91.198	Patient's noncompliance with other medical treatment and regimen for other reason
Z91.89	Other specified personal risk factors, not elsewhere classified
Z92.3	Personal history of irradiation (therapeutic radiation)
Z92.83	Personal history of failed moderate sedation (conscious sedation)
Z92.84	Personal history of unintended awareness under general anesthesia
Z92.89	Personal history of other medical treatment

Nerve Disorders

G50.0	Trigeminal neuralgia
G50.1	Atypical face pain
G50.8	Other disorders of trigeminal nerve
G51.8	Other disorders of facial nerve
G52.1	Disorders of glossopharyngeal nerve
G52.3	Disorder of hypoglossal nerve
G52.8	Disorder of other specified cranial nerve

Sinusitis

J32.0	Chronic maxillary sinusitis
J32.1	Chronic frontal sinusitis
J32.9	Chronic sinusitis, unspecified
R68.2	Dry mouth, unspecified (Not due to Sicca [Sjögren] syndrome)

Other Specified Health Status

Z78.1	Physical restraint status
Z78.9	Other specified health status
Z79.01	Long term (current) use of anticoagulants
Z79.02	Long term (current) use of antithrombotics/antiplatelets
Z79.1	Long term (current) use of non-steroidal anti-inflammatories (NSAID)
Z79.2	Long term (current) use of antibiotics
Z79.4	Long term (current) use of insulin
Z79.51	Long term (current) use of inhaled steroids
Z79.52	Long term (current) use of systemic steroids
Z79.82	Long term (current) use of aspirin
Z79.83	Long term (current) use of bisphosphonates
Z79.84	Long term (current) use of oral hypoglycemic drugs
Z79.891	Long term (current) use of opiate analgesic
Z79.899	Other long term (current) drug therapy

17. Social Determinants

Problems Related to Education and Literacy

Z55.0	Illiteracy and low-level literacy
Z55.1	Schooling unavailable and unattainable
Z55.3	Underachievement in school
Z55.4	Educational maladjustment and discord with teachers and classmates
Z55.8	Other problems related to education and literacy
Z55.9	Problems related to education and literacy, unspecified

Problems Related to Housing and Economic Circumstances

Z59.0	Homelessness
Z59.00	Homelessness unspecified

Z59.01	Sheltered homelessness
Z59.02	Unsheltered homelessness
Z59.1	Inadequate housing
Z59.4	Lack of adequate food and safe drinking water
Z59.41	Food insecurity
Z59.48	Other specified lack of adequate food
Z59.5	Extreme poverty
Z59.6	Low income
Z59.7	Insufficient social insurance and welfare support
Z59.8	Other problems related to housing and economic circumstances

Problems Related to Social Environment

Z60.0	Problems of adjustment to life-cycle transitions
Z60.2	Problems related to living alone
Z60.8	Other problems related to social environment

18. Symptoms and Disorders Pertinent to Orthodontia Cases

Pain

G24.3	Spasmodic toticcollis
G24.4	Idiopathic orofacial dystonia (Orofacial dyskinesia)
G44.1	Vascular headache, not elsewhere classified
G44.201	Tension-type headache, unspecified, intractable
G44.209	Tension-type headache, unspecified, not intractable
G44.211	Episodic tension-type headache, intractable
G44.219	Episodic tension-type headache, not intractable
G44.221	Chronic tension-type headache, intractable
G44.229	Chronic tension-type headache, not intractable
H57.11	Ocular pain, right eye
H57.12	Ocular pain, left eye
H57.13	Ocular pain, bilateral
M79.11	Myalgia of mastication muscle
M79.12	Myalgia of auxiliary muscles, head and neck
M79.18	Myalgia, other site

Migraine

G43.001	Migraine without aura, not intractable, with status migrainosus
G43.009	Migraine without aura, not intractable, without status migrainosus
G43.011	Migraine without aura, intractable, with status migrainosus
G43.019	Migraine without aura, intractable, without status migrainosus
G43.101	Migraine with aura, not intractable, with status migrainosus
G43.109	Migraine with aura, not intractable, without status migrainosus
G43.111	Migraine with aura, not-intractable, with status migrainosus
G43.119	Migraine with aura, intractable, without status migrainosus
G43.701	Chronic migraine without aura, not-intractable, with status migrainosus
G43.719	Chronic migraine without aura, not-intractable, without status migrainosus
G43.801	Other migraine, not intractable, with status migrainosus
G43.809	Other migraine, not intractable, without status migrainosus
G43.811	Other migraine, intractable, with status migrainosus
G43.819	Other migraine, intractable, without status migrainosus
G43.E01	Chronic migraine with aura, not intractable, with status migrainosus
G43.E09	Chronic migraine with aura, not intractable, without status migrainosus
G43.E11	Chronic migraine with aura, intractable, with status migrainosus
G43.E19	Chronic migraine with aura, intractable, without status migrainosus
G44.1	Vascular headache, not elsewhere classified

Ears and Larynx

H92.01	Otalgia, right ear
H92.02	Otalgia, left ear
H92.03	Otalgia, bilateral
H93.11	Tinnitus, right ear
H93.12	Tinnitus, left ear
H93.13	Tinnitus, bilateral
J38.5	Laryngeal spasm

Craniofacial

Q67.0	Congenital facial asymmetry
Q67.4	Other congenital deformities of skull, face and jaw

Q74.0	Other congenital malformations of upper limb(s), including shoulder girdle (Includes Cleidocranial dysostosis)
Q75.001	Craniosynostosis unspecified, unilateral
Q75.002	Craniosynostosis unspecified, bilateral
Q75.009	Craniosynostosis unspecified
Q75.1	Craniofacial dysostosis (Crouzon's disease [syndrome])
Q75.2	Hypertelorism
Q75.3	Macrocephaply
Q75.4	Mandibulofacial dysostosis (Treacher Collins syndrome)
Q75.5	Oculomandibular dysostosis
Q75.8	Other specified malformations of skull and face bones
Q75.9	Congenital malformation of skull and face bones, unspecified
Q87.0	Congenital malformation syndromes predominantly affecting facial appearance (Includes – Acrocephalopolysyndactyly [aka Apert Syndrome and Pfeiffer Syndrome])
Q87.19	Other congenital malformation syndromes predominantly associated with short stature (Includes – Noonan syndrome)

Turners Syndrome

Q96.0	Karyotype 45, X
Q96.2	Karyotype 46, X with abnormal sex chromosome, except iso (Xq)
Q96.3	Mosaicism, 45, X/46, XX or XY
Q96.4	Mosaicism, 45, X/other cell line(s) with abnormal sex chromosome
Q96.8	Other variants of Turner's Syndrome
Q96.9	Turner's Syndrome, unspecified

Other

E22.0	Acromegaly and pituitary gigantism
E23.0	Hypopituitarism (Includes – Isolated deficiency of growth hormone)
G25.3	Myoclonus
R42	Dizziness and giddiness (Includes – Light-headedness)
K00.9	Disorder of tooth development (and eruption), unspecified (aka Disorder of odontogenesis NOS)

Section 4

Alphabetic Index to the CDT Code

Term	Code(s)	Page(s)
A		
A1c testing	D0411	9
Abscess, incision and drainage, all types	D7510, D7511, D7520, D7521	68
Abutments	Also see **Retainers**	
for implants	D6051, D6056, D6057	51
Access opening, closure (for screw-retained implant prosthesis)	D6197	57
Accession of tissue	D0472–D0474	11
Acid etch; part of resin procedure	No separate code	
Adhesives, bonding agents (resin and amalgam bonding agents); part of restorative procedure	No separate code	
Adjunctive General Services (Category of Service)		80–86
Adjunctive pre-diagnostic test	D0431	10
Adjust		
prosthetic appliance	D5992	41
orthodontic retainer	D8681	78
Aesthetic appliance (custom removable)		
fabrication clear plastic temporary	D9938	83, 102
placement clear plastic temporary	D9939	83, 102
Allograft, soft tissue	D4275, D7955	33, 74
Alveoloplasty	D7310, D7311, D7320, D7321	66
Alveolus, fracture	D7670, D7671, D7770, D7771	69, 70
Amalgam restorations	D2140–D2161	18
Amalgam and resin bonding agents (part of restorative procedure)	No separate code	

Term	Code(s)	Page(s)
Analgesia		
inhalation of nitrous oxide	D9230	81
non-intravenous conscious sedation	D9248	81
Anchorage device, temporary		
requiring flap	D7293	65
without flap	D7294	65
screw retained plate requiring flap	D7292	65
Anesthesia		
evaluation for...general	D9219	80
general	D9222, D9223	80, 81
local	D9210, D9215	80
regional	D9211	80
trigeminal division block	D9212	80
Ankyloglossia	See **frenectomy/frenotomy (frenulectomy)**	
Apexification/recalcification	D3351–D3353	25
Apexogenesis	D3222	23
Apically positioned flap	D4245	31
Apicoectomy	D3410–D3473	26
Appliance removal (not by dentist who placed)	D7997	76
Application (hydroxyapatite regeneration medicament)	D2991	21, 93
Appointment		
cancelled	D9987	85
missed	D9986	85
Arthrocentesis	D7870	71
Arthroplasty	D7865	71
Arthroscopy	D7872–D7877	71
Arthrotomy	D7860	71
Assessment of a patient	D0191	5
Athletic mouthguard	D9941	83
Autologous blood concentrate (collection and application)	D7921	72

Term	Code(s)	Page(s)
B		
Bacteriologic studies	D0415	9
Band stabilization	D2976	22, 93
Behavior management	D9920	83
Biologic materials	D4265	32
in conjunction with periradicular surgery	D3431	27
Biopsy		
brush	D7288	65
hard tissue	D7285	65
salivary glands	D7284	64, 100
soft tissue	D7286	65
Bitewing radiographs	D0270–D0274, D0277, D0708	6, 8
Bleaching		
external – per arch	D9972	85
external – per tooth	D9973	85
external – for home application	D9975	85
internal – per tooth	D9974	85
Blood glucose level test	D0412	9
Bone fragment (post-surgical removal)	D9930	83
Bone, harvest of	D7295	65
Bone tissue, excision	D7471–D7490	68
Bonding agents; adhesives (resin and amalgam bonding agents)	No separate code – part of restorative procedure	
Bridge	See **Fixed Partial Dentures**	
Bruxism appliance	D9944–D9946	84
C		
Cancelled appointment	D9987	85
Caries		
arresting medicament application	D1354	14
preventive medicament application	D1355	14
risk assessment	D0601–D0603	10
susceptibility test	D0425	10

Term	Code(s)	Page(s)
adjustments	D5410–D5422	37
complete	D5110–D5120	36
immediate, complete	D5130, D5140	36
implant/abutment supported, complete	D6110, D6111	52
implant/abutment supported, partial	D6112, D6113	52
modification of removable prosthesis following implant surgery	D5875	40
overdenture	D5863–D5866	40
partial	D5211–D5286	36, 37
precision attachment	D5862	40
rebase	D5710–D5721	38
hybrid prosthesis	D5725	38
reline	D5730–D5761	39
repairs, complete and partial	D5511, D5512, D5520, D5611, D5612, D5621, D5622, D5671	38
soft liner	D5765	39
temporary/interim	D5810–D5821	39
Dentures (fixed)		
implant/abutment supported, full	D6114, D6115	52
implant/abutment supported, partial	D6116, D6117	52
implant/abutment supported, interim	D6118, D6119	52, 53
Desensitizing medicament	D9910	83
Desensitizing resin	D9911	83
Destruction of lesion	D7465	67
Diabetes testing (A1c)	D0411	9
Diagnostic (Category of Service)		3–12
Diagnostic casts	D0470	10
Diagnostic imaging		
3D surface scan	D0801–D0804	7
image capture and interpretation	D0210–D0804	5–7
image capture only	D0380–D0389, D0701–D0709	7, 8
interpretation and report only	D0391	8
post processing image or image sets	D0393–D0395	9

Term	Code(s)	Page(s)
Frenectomy/frenotomy (frenulectomy)	D7961–D7962	74
buccal/labial	D7961	74
lingual	D7962	74
Frenuloplasty	D7963	74
Full mouth series (comprehensive; FMX)	D0210, D0709	5, 8

G

Term	Code(s)	Page(s)
Genetic testing		
sample collection	D0422	9
specimen analysis	D0423	9
Gingiva, pericoronal, removal of	D7971	75
Gingival flap	D4240, D4241	30
Gingival Irrigation	D4921	35
Gingivectomy/gingivoplasty	D4210–D4212	29
Glass ionomers (see **resin restorations**)	D2330–D2394	18
Glucose meter – blood level test	D0412	9
Gold foil	D2410–D2430	18
Graft		
bone replacement	D4263, D4264, D6103, D6104, D7953	31, 32, 51, 74
combined connective tissue and pedicle	D4276	33
free soft tissue	D4277, D4278	34
maxillofacial soft/hard tissue	D7955	74
osseous, osteoperiosteal, or cartilage	D7950	73
pedicle soft tissue	D4270	33
periradicular	D3428, D3429	27
sinus augmentation	D7951	73
skin	D7920	72
soft tissue	D4270, D4273	33
connective tissue		
autogenous	D4273, D4283	33
non–autogenous	D4275, D4285	33
synthetic	D7955	74

Term	Code(s)	Page(s)
Guided tissue regeneration (GTR)		
edentulous area	D7956, D7957	74
natural teeth	D4266, D4267	32
per implant	D6106, D6107	51
in conjunction with periradicular surgery	D3432	27
H		
Harvest of bone	D7295	65
Hemisection	D3920	28
Hospital call (hospital or ambulatory surgical center visit)	D9420	82
House call (nursing home visit)	D9410	82
Hemostasis (clot stabilization)	D7922	72
HPV – human papillomavirus (vaccination)	D1781–D1783	16
HSAT (home sleep apnea test)	D9956	87, 103
Hyperplastic tissue, removal of	D7970	74
I		
Images, oral/facial	D0350; D0703	6, 8
Immediate denture		
complete	D5130, D5140	36
partial	D5221–D5224	36, 37
Immunization counseling	D1301	13, 92
Impacted tooth, removal of	D7220–D7241	63
Implant		
abutments	D6056, D6057, D6051	51
chin	D7995	75
endodontic	D3460	27
endosteal/endosseous	D6010	50
eposteal/subperiosteal	D6040	50
interim implant	D6012	50
maintenance	D6080	57
mandible	D7996	76
mini	D6013	50

Term	Code(s)	Page(s)
Interpretation of diagnostic image (different practitioner)	D0391	8
Intraorifice barrier	D3911	28
Intravenous moderate (conscious) sedation/analgesia	D9239, D9243	81
Irrigation (gingival)	D4921	35
J		
Joint reconstruction	D7858	71
K		
No "K" terms		
L		
Labial veneer	D2960–D2962	22
Laser	No separate code – part of dental procedure code that appropriately describes the service provided	
Lateral exostosis	D7471	68
LeFort I	D7946, D7947	73
LeFort II; LeFort III	D7948, D7949	73
Lesions, surgical excision		
intra-osseous lesions	D7440–D7461	67
soft tissue	D7410–D7415, D7465	67
Limited orthodontic treatment	D8010–D8040	77
Localized osteitis/dry socket	D9930	83
M		
Maintenance and cleaning of prosthesis	D5993	41
Malar bone, repair of fracture	D7650, D7660, D7750, D7760	69, 70
Malocclusion, correction of (*see* Orthodontics Category of Service)		
Mandible, fracture of	D7630–D7640, D7730–D7740	69, 70
Marsupialization (odontogenic cyst)	D7509	68
Maryland Bridge (resin bonded fixed prosthesis)		
retainer/abutment	D6545, D6548, D6549	60
pontic	D6210–D6252	59

Term	Code(s)	Page(s)
Maxilla, repair of fracture	D7610–D7620, D7710–D7720	69
Maxillofacial defect	D7955	74
Maxillofacial MRI		
capture and interpretation	D0369	6
image capture (only)	D0385	7
Maxillofacial ultrasound		
capture and interpretation	D0370	7
image capture (only)	D0386	7
Mesial/distal wedge	D4274	33
Metals, classification of		
Metal substructure	D5876	40, 96
Microabrasion, enamel	D9970	85
Microorganisms, culture and sensitivity	D0415	9
Minimal (mild) sedation	D9248	81
Missed appointment	D9986	85
Moderate sedation	D9239, D9243, D9248	81
Molecular test	D0606	10
Moulage, facial	D5911, D5912	42
Mouthguard, athletic	D9941	83
Mucosal abnormalities, pre-diagnostic test	D0431	10
Myotomy	D7856	71
N		
Neoplasms, removal of	D7410–D7465	67
Nightguard	D9944–D9946	84
Nitrous oxide, analgesia	D9230	81
Non-intravenous moderate (conscious) sedation	D9248	81
Non-odontogenic cyst	D7460, D7461	67
Non-resorbable barrier (removal)	D4286	32
Nursing home, (house/extended care facility visit)	D9410	82
Nutritional counseling	D1310	13

Term	Code(s)	Page(s)
Sedation		
evaluation for moderate, deep	D9219	80
deep	D9222, D9223	80, 81
intravenous, moderate (conscious)	D9239, D9243	81
non-intravenous conscious		
minimal (mild)	D9248	81
moderate	D9248	81
Sedative filling	See **Protective Restoration**	
Semi-precision attachment abutment	D6191	52
Semi-precision attachment	D6192	52
Sequestrectomy	D7550	69
Sialodochoplasty	D7982	75
Sialoendoscopy capture and interpretation	D0371	7
Sialography	D0310	6
Sialolithotomy		
non-surgical	D7979	75
surgical	D7980	75
Sign language services, certified	D9990	85
Sinus augmentation		
via lateral open approach	D7951	73
via vertical approach	D7952	73
Sinus perforation, closure	D7261	74
Sinusotomy	D7560	69
Skin graft	D7920	72
Sleep apnea appliance (custom)		
fabrication and placement	D9947, D9954, D9955	87, 103
adjustment	D9948	87
reline	D9953	87
repair	D9949	87
Sleep Apnea Services (Category of Service)		87
Sleep apnea test (home)	D9956	87, 103
Space maintainer	D1510–D1575	14, 15
fixed – bilateral, maxillary	D1516	14

Term	Code(s)	Page(s)
fixed – bilateral, mandibular	D1517	14
removable – bilateral, maxillary	D1526	15
removable – bilateral, mandibular	D1527	15
distal shoe	D1575	15
re-cement or re-bond bilateral, maxillary	D1551	15
re-cement or re-bond unilateral, per quadrant	D1553	15
re-cement or re-bond bilateral, mandibular	D1552	15
removal fixed – unilateral, per quadrant	D1556	15
removal fixed – bilateral, maxillary	D1557	15
removal fixed – bilateral, mandibular	D1558	15
Speech aid		
adult	D5953	47
pediatric	D5952	47
Splinting		
commissure	D5987	41
extra-coronal	D4323	34
intra-coronal	D4322	34
surgical	D5988	48
Stainless steel crown	D2930, D2931, D2933, D2934	21
Stayplate (aka "flipper")	D5820, D5821	39
Stent	D5982	48
Stress breaker	D6940	62
Supra crestal fiberotomy	D7291	65
Surface scan (3D)	D0801–D0804	7
Surgical/ambulatory center	D9420	82
Sustained release therapeutic drug (infiltration of)	D9613	82
Substance use	D1321	14
Surgical access implant body (second stage implant surgery)	D6011	50
Surgical exposure of root surface (without apicoectomy or root resorption repair)	D3501–D3503	26, 27
Surgical placement of craniofacial implant	D7993	75

Term	Code(s)	Page(s)
Tobacco counseling	D1320	13
Tomographic survey	D0322	6
Tomosynthesis		
image capture with interpretation	D0372–D0374	7, 89
image capture only	D0387–D0389	8, 89
Tongue thrusting appliance	D8210, D8220	78
Tooth, natural		
caries susceptibility test	D0425	10
extraction	D7111, D7140, D7210–D7250	63, 64
impacted, removal of	D7220–D7241	63
intentional re-implantation	D3470	27
pulp vitality test	D0460	10
re-implantation, evulsed/displaced	D7270	64
access of an unerupted tooth (surgical)	D7280	64
surgical repositioning	D7290	65
transplantation	D7272	64
Tooth, reattach fragment	D2921	21
Tooth surface codes		17
Topical medicament carrier	D5991	49
Torus, removal of		
mandibularis	D7473	68
palatinus	D7472	68
Tracheotomy, emergency	D7990	75
Transplantation, tooth	D7272	64
Transseptal fiberotomy	D7291	65
Trismus appliance	D5937	48
Tuberosity		
fibrous	D7972	75
osseous (reduction, surgical)	D7485	68
Tumors, removal of	D7440–D7465	67

U

Term	Code(s)	Page(s)
Un-erupted tooth, access	D7280	64
Unilateral removable partial denture	D5282–5286	37

Section 5

Numeric Index to the CDT Code

CDT Category		Code Entry Change (when applicable)		CDT Category		Code Entry Change (when applicable)	
Code	Page	Addition **Revision** Deletion **Editorial**	Page	Code	Page	Addition **Revision** Deletion **Editorial**	Page
I. Diagnostic				D0350	6		
D0120	3			D0364	6		
D0140	3			D0365	6		
D0145	3			D0366	6		
D0150	4			D0367	6		
D0160	4			D0368	6		
D0170	4			D0369	6		
D0171	4			D0370	7		
D0180	5			D0371	7		
D0190	5			D0372	7		
D0191	5			D0373	7		
D0210	5			D0374	7		
D0220	5			D0380	7		
D0230	5			D0381	7		
D0240	5			D0382	7		
D0250	5			D0383	7		
D0251	6			D0384	7		
D0270	6			D0385	7		
D0272	6			D0386	7		
D0273	6			D0387	8		
D0274	6			D0388	8		
D0277	6			D0389	8		
D0310	6			D0391	8		
D0320	6			D0393	9		
D0321	6			D0394	9		
D0322	6			D0395	9		
D0330	6			D0396	9	Addition	91
D0340	6			D0411	9		

CDT Category		Code Entry Change (when applicable)		CDT Category		Code Entry Change (when applicable)	
Code	Page	Addition Revision Deletion Editorial	Page	Code	Page	Addition Revision Deletion Editorial	Page
D0412	9			D0703	8		
D0414	9			D0705	8		
D0415	9			D0706	8		
D0416	9			D0707	8		
D0417	9			D0708	8		
D0418	9			D0709	8		
D0419	9			D0801	7		
D0422	9			D0802	7		
D0423	10			D0803	7		
D0425	10			D0804	7		
D0431	10			D0999	12		
D0460	10			**II. Preventive**			
D0470	10			D1110	13		
D0472	11			D1120	13		
D0473	11			D1206	13		
D0474	11			D1208	13		
D0475	11			D1301	13	Addition	92
D0476	11			D1310	13		
D0477	11			D1320	13		
D0478	12			D1321	14		
D0479	12			D1330	14		
D0480	11			D1351	14		
D0481	12			D1352	14		
D0482	12			D1353	14		
D0483	12			D1354	14		
D0484	12			D1355	14		
D0485	12			D1510	14		
D0486	11			D1516	14		
D0502	12			D1517	14		
D0600	10			D1520	15		
D0601	10			D1526	15		
D0602	10			D1527	15		
D0603	10			D1551	15		
D0604	10			D1552	15		
D0605	10			D1553	15		
D0606	10			D1556	15		
D0701	8			D1557	15		
D0702	8			D1558	15		

CDT Category		Code Entry Change (when applicable)		CDT Category		Code Entry Change (when applicable)	
Code	Page	Addition **Revision** Deletion Editorial	Page	Code	Page	Addition **Revision** Deletion Editorial	Page
D1575	15			D2542	19		
D1701	15			D2543	19		
D1702	15			D2544	19		
D1703	15			D2610	19		
D1704	15			D2620	19		
D1705	15			D2630	19		
D1706	15			D2642	19		
D1707	15			D2643	19		
D1708	16			D2644	19		
D1709	16			D2650	19		
D1710	16			D2651	19		
D1711	16			D2652	19		
D1712	16			D2662	19		
D1713	16			D2663	19		
D1714	16			D2664	19		
D1781	16			D2710	20		
D1782	16			D2712	20		
D1783	16			D2720	20		
D1999	16			D2721	20		
III. Restorative				D2722	20		
D2140	18			D2740	20		
D2150	18			D2750	20		
D2160	18			D2751	20		
D2161	18			D2752	20		
D2330	18			D2753	20		
D2331	18			D2780	20		
D2332	18			D2781	20		
D2335	18	**Revision**	93	D2782	20		
D2390	18			D2783	20		
D2391	18			D2790	20		
D2392	18			D2791	20		
D2393	18			D2792	20		
D2394	18			D2794	20		
D2410	18			D2799	20		
D2420	18			D2910	21		
D2430	18			D2915	21		
D2510	19			D2920	21		
D2520	19			D2921	21		
D2530	19			D2928	21		

Numeric Index to the CDT Code

CDT Category		Code Entry Change (when applicable)		CDT Category		Code Entry Change (when applicable)	
Code	Page	Addition **Revision** Deletion Editorial	Page	Code	Page	Addition **Revision** Deletion Editorial	Page
D2929	21			D3310	24		
D2930	21			D3320	24		
D2931	21			D3330	24		
D2932	21			D3331	24		
D2933	21			D3332	24		
D2934	21			D3333	24		
D2940	21			D3346	25		
D2941	21			D3347	25		
D2949	21			D3348	25		
D2950	21			D3351	25		
D2951	21			D3352	25		
D2952	22			D3353	25		
D2953	22			D3355	25		
D2954	22			D3356	25		
D2955	22			D3357	25		
D2957	22			D3410	26		
D2960	22			D3421	26		
D2961	22			D3425	26		
D2962	22			D3426	26		
D2971	22			D3428	27		
D2975	22			D3429	27		
D2976	22	Addition	93	D3430	27		
D2980	22			D3431	27		
D2981	22			D3432	27		
D2982	22			D3450	27		
D2983	22			D3460	27		
D2989	20	Addition	93	D3470	27		
D2990	20			D3471	26		
D2991	21	Addition	93	D3472	26		
D2999	22			D3473	26		
IV. Endodontics				D3501	26		
D3110	23			D3502	27		
D3120	23			D3503	27		
D3220	23			D3910	28		
D3221	23			D3911	28		
D3222	23			D3920	28		
D3230	24			D3921	28		
D3240	24			D3950	28		
				D3999	28		

CDT Category		Code Entry Change (when applicable)		CDT Category		Code Entry Change (when applicable)	
Code	Page	Addition Revision Deletion Editorial	Page	Code	Page	Addition Revision Deletion Editorial	Page
V. Periododontics				VI. Prosthodontics (removable)			
D4210	29			D5110	36		
D4211	29			D5120	36		
D4212	29			D5130	36		
D4230	30			D5140	36		
D4231	30			D5211	36		
D4240	30			D5212	36		
D4241	30			D5213	36		
D4245	31			D5214	36		
D4249	31			D5221	36		
D4260	31			D5222	37		
D4261	31			D5223	37		
D4263	31			D5224	37		
D4264	32			D5225	36		
D4265	32			D5226	36		
D4266	32			D5227	37		
D4267	32			D5228	37		
D4268	32			D5282	37		
D4270	33			D5283	37		
D4273	33			D5284	37		
D4274	33			D5286	37		
D4275	33			D5410	37		
D4276	33			D5411	37		
D4277	34			D5421	37		
D4278	34			D5422	37		
D4283	33			D5511	38		
D4285	33			D5512	38		
D4286	32			D5520	38		
D4322	34			D5611	38		
D4323	34			D5612	38		
D4341	34			D5621	38		
D4342	34			D5622	38		
D4346	35			D5630	38		
D4355	35			D5640	38		
D4381	35			D5650	38		
D4910	35			D5660	38		
D4920	35			D5670	38		
D4921	35			D5671	38		
D4999	35			D5710	38		

CDT Category		Code Entry Change (when applicable)	
Code	Page	Addition **Revision** Deletion Editorial	Page
D5711	38		
D5720	38		
D5721	38		
D5725	38		
D5730	39		
D5731	39		
D5740	39		
D5741	39		
D5750	39		
D5751	39		
D5760	39		
D5761	39		
D5765	39		
D5810	39		
D5811	39		
D5820	39		
D5821	39		
D5850	39		
D5851	39		
D5862	40		
D5863	40		
D5864	40		
D5865	40		
D5866	40		
D5867	40		
D5875	40		
D5876	40	**Revision**	96
D5899	40		
VII. Maxillofacial Prosthetics			
D5911	42		
D5912	42		
D5913	43		
D5914	41		
D5915	45		
D5916	45		
D5919	42		
D5922	44		
D5923	45		
D5924	41		

CDT Category		Code Entry Change (when applicable)	
Code	Page	Addition **Revision** Deletion Editorial	Page
D5925	41		
D5926	43		
D5927	41		
D5928	46		
D5929	42		
D5931	45		
D5932	44		
D5933	44		
D5934	43		
D5935	43		
D5936	44		
D5937	48		
D5951	42		
D5952	47		
D5953	47		
D5954	46		
D5955	46		
D5958	46		
D5959	46		
D5960	47		
D5982	48		
D5983	49		
D5984	47		
D5985	46		
D5986	48		
D5987	41		
D5988	48		
D5991	49		
D5992	41		
D5993	41		
D5995	49		
D5996	49		
D5999	49		
VIII. Implant Services			
D6010	50		
D6011	50		
D6012	50		
D6013	50		
D6040	50		

CDT Category		Code Entry Change (when applicable)		CDT Category		Code Entry Change (when applicable)	
Code	Page	Addition **Revision** Deletion Editorial	Page	Code	Page	Addition **Revision** Deletion Editorial	Page
D6050	50			D6094	53		
D6051	51			D6095	57		
D6055	51			D6096	57		
D6056	51			D6097	53		
D6057	51			D6098	56		
D6058	53			D6099	56		
D6059	53			D6100	50		
D6060	53			D6101	51		
D6061	53			D6102	51		
D6062	53			D6103	51		
D6063	53			D6104	51		
D6064	53			D6105	51		
D6065	54			D6106	51		
D6066	54			D6107	51		
D6067	54			D6110	52		
D6068	55			D6111	52		
D6069	55			D6112	52		
D6070	55			D6113	52		
D6071	55			D6114	52		
D6072	55			D6115	52		
D6073	55			D6116	52		
D6074	55			D6117	52		
D6075	56			D6118	52		
D6076	56			D6119	52		
D6077	56			D6120	56		
D6080	57			D6121	56		
D6081	57			D6122	56		
D6082	54			D6123	56		
D6083	54			D6190	50		
D6084	54			D6191	52		
D6085	57			D6192	52		
D6086	54			D6194	55		
D6087	54			D6195	55		
D6088	54			D6197	57		
D6089	57	Addition	98	D6198	58		
D6090	57			D6199	58		
D6091	57			**IX. Prosthodontics, Fixed**			
D6092	57			D6205	59		
D6093	57			D6210	59		

CDT Category		Code Entry Change (when applicable)		CDT Category		Code Entry Change (when applicable)	
Code	Page	Addition Revision Deletion Editorial	Page	Code	Page	Addition Revision Deletion Editorial	Page
D6211	59			D6751	61		
D6212	59			D6752	61		
D6214	59			D6753	61		
D6240	59			D6780	61		
D6241	59			D6781	61		
D6242	59			D6782	61		
D6243	59			D6783	61		
D6245	59			D6784	61		
D6250	59			D6790	61		
D6251	59			D6791	61		
D6252	59			D6792	61		
D6253	59			D6793	61		
D6545	60			D6794	61		
D6548	60			D6920	62		
D6549	60			D6930	62		
D6600	60			D6940	62		
D6601	60			D6950	62		
D6602	60			D6980	62		
D6603	60			D6985	62		
D6604	60			D6999	62		
D6605	60			X. Oral & Maxillofacial Surgery			
D6606	60			D7111	63		
D6607	60			D7140	63		
D6608	60			D7210	63		
D6609	60			D7220	63		
D6610	60			D7230	63		
D6611	60			D7240	63		
D6612	60			D7241	63		
D6613	60			D7250	64		
D6614	60			D7251	64		
D6615	60			D7260	64		
D6624	60			D7261	64		
D6634	60			D7270	64		
D6710	61			D7272	64		
D6720	61			D7280	64		
D6721	61			D7282	64		
D6722	61			D7283	64		
D6740	61			D7284	64	Addition	100
D6750	61			D7285	65		

CDT Category		Code Entry Change (when applicable)		CDT Category		Code Entry Change (when applicable)	
Code	Page	Addition Revision Deletion Editorial	Page	Code	Page	Addition Revision Deletion Editorial	Page
D7286	65			D7510	68		
D7287	65			D7511	68		
D7288	65			D7520	68		
D7290	65			D7521	68		
D7291	65			D7530	68		
D7292	65			D7540	68		
D7293	65			D7550	69		
D7294	65			D7560	69		
D7295	65			D7610	69		
D7296	66			D7620	69		
D7297	66			D7630	69		
D7298	65			D7640	69		
D7299	65			D7650	69		
D7300	65			D7660	69		
D7310	66			D7670	69		
D7311	66			D7671	69		
D7320	66			D7680	69		
D7321	66			D7710	69		
D7340	67			D7720	69		
D7350	67			D7730	69		
D7410	67			D7740	70		
D7411	67			D7750	70		
D7412	67			D7760	70		
D7413	67			D7770	70		
D7414	67			D7771	70		
D7415	67			D7780	70		
D7440	67			D7810	70		
D7441	67			D7820	70		
D7450	67			D7830	70		
D7451	67			D7840	70		
D7460	67			D7850	70		
D7461	67			D7852	70		
D7465	67			D7854	70		
D7471	68			D7856	71		
D7472	68			D7858	71		
D7473	68			D7860	71		
D7485	68			D7865	71		
D7490	68			D7870	71		
D7509	68			D7871	71		

CDT Category		Code Entry Change (when applicable)		CDT Category		Code Entry Change (when applicable)	
Code	Page	Addition **Revision** Deletion Editorial	Page	Code	Page	Addition **Revision** Deletion Editorial	Page
D7872	71			D7979	75		
D7873	71			D7980	75		
D7874	71			D7981	75		
D7875	71			D7982	75		
D7876	71			D7983	75		
D7877	71			D7990	75		
D7880	71			D7991	75		
D7881	71			D7993	75		
D7899	72			D7994	75		
D7910	72			D7995	75		
D7911	72			D7996	76		
D7912	72			D7997	76		
D7920	72			D7998	76		
D7921	72			D7999	76		
D7922	72			**XI. Orthodontics**			
D7939	72	Addition	100	D8010	77		
D7940	72			D8020	77		
D7941	72			D8030	77		
D7943	72			D8040	77		
D7944	73			D8070	78		
D7945	73			D8080	78		
D7946	73			D8090	78		
D7947	73			D8210	78		
D7948	73			D8220	78		
D7949	73			D8660	78		
D7950	73			D8670	78		
D7951	73			D8680	78		
D7952	73			D8681	78		
D7953	74			D8695	78		
D7955	74			D8696	79		
D7956	74			D8697	79		
D7957	74			D8698	79		
D7961	74			D8699	79		
D7962	74			D8701	79		
D7963	74			D8702	79		
D7970	74			D8703	79		
D7971	75			D8704	79		
D7972	75			D8999	79		

CDT Category		Code Entry Change (when applicable)		CDT Category		Code Entry Change (when applicable)	
Code	Page	Addition Revision Deletion Editorial	Page	Code	Page	Addition Revision Deletion Editorial	Page
XII. Adjunctive General Services				D9942	84		
D9110	80			D9943	84		
D9120	80			D9944	84		
D9130	80			D9945	84		
D9210	80			D9946	84		
D9211	80			D9950	84		
D9212	80			D9951	84		
D9215	80			D9952	84		
D9219	80			D9961	85		
D9222	80			D9970	85		
D9223	81			D9971	85		
D9230	81			D9972	85		
D9239	81			D9973	85		
D9243	81			D9974	85		
D9248	81			D9975	85		
D9310	81			D9985	85		
D9311	81			D9986	85		
D9410	82			D9987	85		
D9420	82			D9990	85		
D9430	82			D9991	85		
D9440	82			D9992	85		
D9450	82			D9993	85		
D9610	82			D9994	86		
D9612	82			D9995	86		
D9613	82			D9996	86		
D9630	82			D9997	86		
D9910	83			D9999	86		
D9911	83			XIII. Sleep Apnea Services			
D9912	83			D9947	87		
D9920	83			D9948	87		
D9930	83			D9949	87		
D9932	83			D9953	87		
D9933	83			D9954	87	Addition	103
D9934	83			D9955	87	Addition	103
D9935	83			D9956	87	Addition	103
D9938	83	Addition	102	D9957	87	Addition	103
D9939	83	Addition	102				
D9941	83						

Get More Out of Coding with the
CDT 2024 App

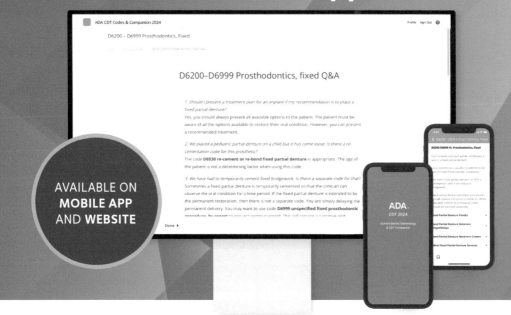

AVAILABLE ON MOBILE APP AND WEBSITE

CDT 2024 App gives you all the information from *CDT 2024* and the *CDT 2024 Coding Companion* in one digital resource. The app allows for easy searching of codes, descriptors, coding examples and more. Look up a code descriptor from a personal device or review a coding scenario right on your desktop, right when you need it.

Features:

- For use on iPhone, Android, tablet or desktop computer—any web-enabled device
- Developed by the ADA, the official source for CDT codes
- Includes CDT codes for 2024 and 2023 plus complete descriptors
- Includes content from the *CDT 2024 Companion*
- Includes ICD-10-CM codes applicable to dentistry

Guess what? The *CDT 2024 App* is already included in your CDT purchase. Find the instructions to access the app on the inside of the front cover of this book.

ADA American Dental Association®

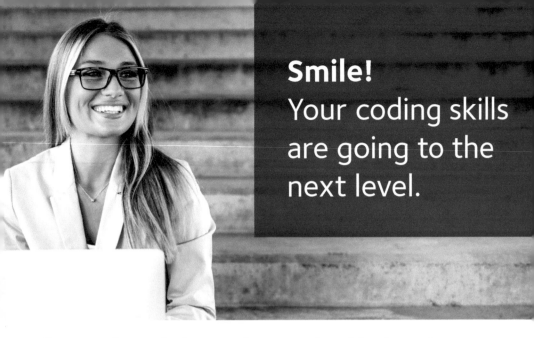

Smile!
Your coding skills are going to the next level.

Take your knowledge to the next level by learning how to use codes in practice.

Mastery of ADA's CDT codes will make you a more valuable asset to the team and practice. Increase your coding skills and complete the **ADA Dental Coding Certificate: Assessment-Based CDT Program**. It helps new and experienced staff members achieve coding proficiency and helps the dental office run more smoothly.

Participants will:
- Gain thorough knowledge of coding terms and tools
- Understand dental procedure codes and how to apply them
- Accurately complete the ADA Dental Claim Form
- Use the *CDT 2024* and *CDT Companion* books correctly

As the official source for CDT® codes, the ADA has answered thousands of questions over the years. When dental teams have questions, we have the answers. Take advantage of our expertise and get up to code today!

Participants will earn 4 CE hours after successfully passing the online assessment. The course is available either with or without CDT books.

ADA American Dental Association®